Ensuring Safe Food

From Production to Consumption

Committee to Ensure Safe Food from Production to Consumption

INSTITUTE OF MEDICINE

NATIONAL RESEARCH COUNCIL

NATIONAL ACADEMY PRESS
Washington, D.C. 1998

ect of this report was approved by the Governing Board of the National Research Council, whose members are drawn from the councils of the National Academy of Sciences, the National Academy of Engineering, and the Institute of Medicine. The members of the committee responsible for the report were chosen for their special competences and with regard for appropriate balance.

The National Academy of Sciences is a private, nonprofit, self-perpetuating society of distinguished scholars engaged in scientific and engineering research, dedicated to the furtherance of science and technology and to their use for the general welfare. Upon the authority of the charter granted to it by the Congress in 1863, the Academy has a mandate that requires it to advise the federal government on scientific and technical matters. Dr. Bruce Alberts is president of the National Academy of Sciences.

The National Academy of Engineering was established in 1964, under the charter of the National Academy of Sciences, as a parallel organization of outstanding engineers. It is autonomous in its administration and in the selection of its members, sharing with the National Academy of Sciences the responsibility for advising the federal government. The National Academy of Engineering also sponsors engineering programs aimed at meeting national needs, encourages education and research, and recognizes the superior achievements of engineers. Dr. William A. Wulf is president of the National Academy of Engineering.

The Institute of Medicine was established in 1970 by the National Academy of Sciences to enlist distinguished members of the appropriate professions in the examination of policy matters pertaining to the health of the public. In this, the Institute acts under both the Academy's 1863 congressional charter responsibility to be an adviser to the federal government and its own initiative in identifying issues of medical care, research, and education. Dr. Kenneth I. Shine is president of the Institute of Medicine.

The National Research Council was organized by the National Academy of Sciences in 1916 to link the broad community of science and technology with the Academy's purposes of furthering knowledge and advising the federal government. Functioning in accordance with general policies determined by the Academy, the Council has become the principal operating agency of both the National Academy of Sciences and the National Academy of Engineering in providing services to the government, the public, and the scientific and engineering communities. The Council is administered jointly by both Academies and the Institute of Medicine. Dr. Bruce Alberts and Dr. William A. Wulf are chairman and vice-chairman, respectively, of the National Research Council.

This material is based upon work supported by the U.S. Department of Agriculture, Agricultural Research Service, under Agreement No. 59-0790-8-013. Any opinions, findings, conclusions, or recommendations expressed in this publication are those of the author and do not necessarily reflect the view of the U.S. Department of Agriculture.

Library of Congress Cataloging-in-Publication Data 98-86932
Internation Standard Book No: 0-309-06559-3

This report is available for sale from the National Academy Press, 2101 Constitution Avenue, N.W., Box 285, Washington, DC 20055, Call (800) 624-6242 or (202) 334-3313 (in the Washington metropolitan area), or visit the NAP's on-line bookstore at **http://www.nap.edu**.

COMMITTEE TO ENSURE SAFE FOOD FROM PRODUCTION TO CONSUMPTION

JOHN C. BAILAR III* (*Chair*), Department of Health Studies, The University of Chicago, Illinois

CAROLE A. BISOGNI, Division of Nutritional Sciences, Cornell University, Ithaca, New York

DAVID L. CALL, Retired, College of Agriculture and Life Sciences, Cornell University, Ithaca, New York

MARSHA N. COHEN, Hastings College of the Law, University of California, San Francisco

MICHAEL P. DOYLE, Center for Food Safety and Quality Enhancement, University of Georgia, Griffin

DELIA A. HAMMOCK, Good Housekeeping Institute, New York

LONNIE J. KING, College of Veterinary Medicine, Michigan State University, East Lansing

GILBERT A. LEVEILLE, Leveille Associates, Denville, New Jersey

RICHARD A. MERRILL,* University of Virginia School of Law, Charlottesville, Virginia

SANFORD A. MILLER, Graduate School of Biomedical Sciences, University of Texas Health Science Center, San Antonio

HARLEY W. MOON,† Veterinary Medical Research Institute, Iowa State University, Ames

MICHAEL T. OSTERHOLM, Minnesota Department of Health, Minneapolis

THOMAS D. TRAUTMAN, General Mills, Minneapolis, Minnesota

Staff

ALLISON A. YATES, Study Director
CHARLOTTE KIRK BAER, Senior Program Officer
SANDRA A. SCHLICKER, Senior Program Officer
ELISABETH REESE, Research Associate
KATHERINE J. GORTON, Policy Intern
GAIL E. SPEARS, Administrative Assistant
SHIRLEY B. THATCHER, Administrative Assistant
GERALDINE KENNEDO, Project Assistant
MELINDA SIMONS, Project Assistant

---

*Member, Institute of Medicine.

† Member, National Academy of Sciences.

FOOD SAFETY OVERSIGHT COMMISSION

DONALD KENNEDY (*Chair*),†* Institute for International Studies, Stanford University, California
DALE E. BAUMAN,† Cornell University, Ithaca, New York
FERGUS M. CLYDESDALE, University of Massachusetts at Amherst
JOHANNA T. DWYER, Tufts Medical School and School of Nutrition Science and Policy, New England Medical Center, Boston, Massachusetts
JOHN W. ERDMAN, Jr., College of Agriculture, University of Illinois at Urbana-Champaign
CUTBERTO GARZA, Cornell University, Ithaca, New York
GEORGE R. HALLBERG, The Cadmus Group, Inc., Waltham, Masssachusetts
JOHN W. SUTTIE,† University of Wisconsin-Madison
BAILUS WALKER, Jr.,* Howard University Cancer Center, Washington, DC

Staff

PAUL GILMAN, Executive Director, Board on Agriculture
KAREN HEIN, Executive Officer, Institute of Medicine
MICHAEL J. PHILLIPS, Director, Board on Agriculture
ALLISON A. YATES, Director, Food and Nutrition Board

---

*Member, Institute of Medicine.
†Member, National Academy of Sciences.

Preface

Protecting the food supply from harmful agents and thus promoting the public health is an important activity of government. The current system for food safety in the United States is a complex and multi-layered activity that depends on multiple players that include the federal government, state governments, local governments, universities, the news media, and, of course, the public itself, both as preparers and handlers of food and as consumers. These varied roles which each segment plays in food safety, with their many complexities and charges, must be integrated within the equally complex and changing system of the food supply from production to final consumption. Though the federal roles of guidance, research, surveillance, enforcement, and education are extremely important, they represent only one part of the food safety system.

Given the size and complexity of this multi-faceted system, it is not unexpected that new information and new concerns often emerge. Many are due to advances in science or to changes in food production and consumption patterns. The system itself must then change if it is to maintain effective vigilance over the safety of the food supply. Congress has acted to strengthen the federal role as the primary agent for integration of activities related to food safety. Many components of the federal food safety system determined by Congress have been relatively unchanged over the last few decades, and concerns have come forward that major changes may be required.

At the request of Congress, and in light of the emerging food safety concerns and many recent proposals recommending change, the Agricultural Research Service of the United States Department of Agriculture asked the National Academy of Sciences (NAS) in late 1997 to 1) determine the scientific basis of an effective food safety system, 2) assess the effectiveness of the current food safety system in the United States, 3) identify scientific needs and gaps within the current system, and 4) provide recommendations on scientific and organizational changes in federal food safety activity needed to ensure an effective science-based food safety system.

The Committee to Ensure Safe Food from Production to Consumption was formed by the Institute of Medicine (IOM) and National Research Council (NRC) to do the evaluation in response to this request. The committee reviewed mechanisms now in place at the federal level to ensure safe food, assessed the extent to which they are effective in addressing food safety issues from production to consumption, and developed recommendations about changes needed to move toward a more effective food safety system. This volume reports the deliberations, conclusions, and recommendations of the committee.

The IOM and the NRC also formed an oversight commission composed of members from the Food and Nutrition Board, the Board on Agriculture, and the Board on Environmental Studies and Toxicology of the Commission on Life Sciences. The chair, Donald Kennedy, is a member of both IOM and of NAS. The role of the Commission was to nominate a committee whose expertise would be appropriately balanced for a study of this scope and complexity. The multidisciplinary group included experts in public health, epidemiology, food science, food microbiology, production agriculture, veterinary medicine, food technology, food regulatory law, consumer protection, consumer education, and media communications. In addition, five members of the 13 member committee held previous positions in federal agencies involved in food safety, three were from the food industry, and two from the agriculture/aquaculture industry. And, of course, all committee members are frequent consumers of food (see Appendix G for biographical sketches of each committee member).

The committee held three meetings during its short period of deliberations. The first meeting, held March 23 to 25, 1998, included an open meeting to hear from the federal agencies most involved with food safety and from Dr. Ed Knipling, Associate Administrator of ARS/USDA who served as the project officer for the study. Representatives from each agency were asked to discuss the mission of their agency and its involvement in regulatory efforts, and to provide the agency budget for key activities related to food safety (see Appendix E).

The second meeting, held April 28 to May 1, 1998, was held in conjunction with an open meeting to which individuals representing many of the major organizations with interests related to food safety presented their responses to three questions:

1) What works well in the current US food safety system?
2) What changes would lead to a more effective food safety system?
3) What types of changes would be detrimental to an effective food safety system?

A summary of the major points made by invited participants during the second workshop appears as Appendix D in the report.

The final meeting of the committee, held June 12-14, 1998, did not include an open portion. At this meeting, the committee finished its major deliberations related to the report and finalized its recommendations.

The Executive Summary presents the committee's principal findings and recommendations from its review of the four areas it was charged to consider. Chapter 1 provides an introduction to the issues and concerns related to food safety, including a brief history of food safety legislation since the early 1900's. Chapter 2 describes the current food safety system, with special attention to the federal role. Public health hazards resulting from the changing nature of pathogens and other toxicants are discussed in Chapter 3. Chapter 4 presents the committee's judgment regarding the attributes of a model food safety system. Chapter 5 compares the current federal system with the model system and identifies gaps. Chapter 6 includes the major conclusions and recommendations of the committee regarding changes needed in approaches and organizational structure to move toward a more effective food safety system. The appendices include reports and information related to the overall issues: Appendix A includes organizational charts, which identify the various components of the federal governments with functions related to food safety; Appendix B includes a recently released report from the Congressional Research Service outlining past recommendations for organizational change in food safety at the federal level; Appendix C includes the executive summary from *Food Safety from Farm to Table: A National Food-Safety Initiative;* Appendix D is a summary of points presented to the committee at their open meeting in April by representatives of various groups with interests in food safety, Appendix E includes information provided by federal agencies on levels of funding attributed to the major components of food safety for the years 1995-98, and Appendix F acknowledges the many individuals who assisted the committee by providing comments and materials in the information-gathering phase of the study.

This report has been reviewed in draft form by individuals chosen for their diverse perspectives and technical expertise, in accordance with procedures approved by the NRC Report Review Committee. The purpose of this independent review is to provide candid and critical comments that will assist the IOM and the NRC in making the published report as sound as possible and to ensure that the report meets institutional standards for objectivity, evidence, and responsiveness to the study charge. The content of the final report is the responsibility of the IOM, NRC, and the study committee, and not the responsibility of the reviewers. The review comments and draft manuscript remain confidential to protect the integrity of the deliberative process. The Committee to Ensure Safe Food From Production to Consumption thanks the following individuals, who are neither officials nor employees of the IOM or the NRC, for their participation in the review of this report: Francis F. Busta, University of Minnesota; Lester Crawford, Georgetown University; Bernard D. Goldstein, UMDNJ-Robert Wood Johnson Medical School; Ray Hankes,

Preferred Stock Genetic, Inc.; Carol Tucker Foreman, Foreman, Heiderpriem and Mager, Inc.; Cynthia M. Harris, Florida A&M University; Donald Hornig, Harvard University; Malden Nesheim, Cornell University; Stuart E. Richardson, California Department of Health Services; Mark Silbergeld, Consumers Union; and Bruce Stillings, Food & Agriculture Consultants. While the individuals listed above have provided many constructive comments and suggestions, it must be emphasized that responsibility for the final content of this report rests entirely with the authoring committee, the IOM, and the NRC.

On behalf of the committee, it is a pleasure to thank Allison Yates, study director, senior staff officers Charlotte Kirk Baer and Sandra Schlicker, research associate Elisabeth Reese, IOM policy intern Kate Gorton, and project assistants Geraldine Kennedo and Melinda Simons. Their efforts were essential to the timely conclusion of our mission. Additionally, the committee thanks Michael Phillips for his assistance as director of the Board on Agriculture and Shirley Thatcher, his administrative assistant, and Norman Grossblatt of the Commission on Life Sciences for his valued editorial assistance early in the development of the report. We thank Michael A. Edington from the IOM Reports and Information Office for assistance in the production of the report and Claudia Carl, who managed the report review process. We also thank all who provided comments to the committee during the course of its deliberations.

It is a pleasure also to record my personal thanks to the committee itself, which accomplished a prodigious amount of high-quality analysis and interpretation in a very short time.

John C. Bailar III,
Chair,
Committee to Ensure Safe Food from Production to Consumption

Contents

EXECUTIVE SUMMARY   1

1   INTRODUCTION AND BACKGROUND   17
Changes in the US Food System and Their Effects on Food Safety, 18
Scope of the Food Safety Problem, 20
History of US Food Safety Regulation, 21
The Committee and Its Charge, 23

2   THE CURRENT US FOOD SAFETY SYSTEM   25
Regulation, 26
     Federal Regulatory Programs, 26
     State and Local Regulatory Systems, 28
     HACCP Systems, 29
     Voluntary Efforts, 31
     Liability, 33
Surveillance, 34
     Human and Animal Disease, 34
     Chemical Residues and Environmental Contaminants, 36
Technical Guidance and Education, 38
     Government Activities, 38
     Private Efforts, 39
Consumer Responsibility and Perceptions, 39

The Role of Media-Government Partnerships in Food Safety
        Education, 42
Research and Development, 43
    Federal Research Activities, 43
    Application of New Technology, 45
International Dimensions, 46
    Food Safety Efforts of Other Countries, 46
    US Regulation of Imported Foods, 47
Summary Findings: The Current US System for Food Safety, 49

3   THE CHANGING NATURE OF FOOD HAZARDS: CAUSE FOR
     INCREASING CONCERN   51
Changes that Affect the Epidemiology of Foodborne Disease, 51
    Diet, 52
    Commercial Food Services, 54
    Methods of Production and Distribution, 54
    New or Re-emerging Infectious Foodborne Agents, 55
    Populations at High Risk for Severe or Fatal Foodborne Disease, 56
Changes in Chemical Hazards Associated with the Food Supply, 57
    New Food Components, 58
    New Food Technologies, 59
    New or Re-emerging Toxic Agents, 59
    Physical Hazards, 60
Summary Findings: The Changing Nature of Food Hazards, 61

4   WHAT CONSTITUTES AN EFFECTIVE FOOD
     SAFETY SYSTEM?   63
The Mission of the System, 63
General Attributes of the System, 65
The Importance of Partnering, 67
The Roles of Government Partners, 67
    A Science-Based Foundation Using Risk Analysis, 68
    Adequate Surveillance and Monitoring, 69
    Focused Education and Research, 69
    Effective and Consistent Regulation and Enforcement, 71
    Response and Adaptation to New Technology and Changing Consumer
        Needs, 71
    Human and Financial Resources, 72
The Roles of Private-Sector Partners, 73
    Producers, 73
    Processors, Marketers, and Distributors, 74
The Role of the Consumer, 75
The Role of Other Partners, 76
A Dynamic Interdependence, 77
Summary Findings: An Effective Food Safety System, 78

5 WHERE CURRENT US FOOD SAFETY ACTIVITIES FALL SHORT 79

Inadequate Application of Science, 80

Research Funding Levels, 81

Recent Efforts to Improve Research, 82

Inadequate Use of Risk Assessment, 82

Insufficient Information, 83

HACCP Systems and Their Limitations, 84

Absence of Focused Leadership, 85

Statutory Limitations, 85

Lack of Coordination, 87

Deficiencies in Regulation of Imported Food, 89

Summary Findings: Where the US Food Safety System Falls Short, 90

6 CONCLUSIONS AND RECOMMENDATIONS 91

Scientific Recommendations, 92

Rationale for Recommendations Related to a Science-Based System, 95

Role of Risk Analysis, 96

Resources Required for Research, 96

Recommendations to Implement a Science-Based System Through Organizational Changes, 97

Rationale for Organizational Recommendations, 98

Centralized and Unified Federal Framework, 98

Integration of Food Safety Efforts, 99

REFERENCES 101

APPENDIXES 105

A Glossary and Organizational Framework for Current Food Safety System, 105

B CRS Report for Congress, *Food Safety: Recommendations for Changes in the Organization of Federal Food Safety Responsibilities, 1949-1997*, 115

C Executive Summary: *Food Safety From Farm to Table: A National Food-Safety Initiative*, 161

D Summary of Comments and Testimony from Workshop (April 29-30, 1998) and Agenda, 169

E Federal Food Safety Budget Information, 181

F Acknowledgments, 185

G Committee Biographical Sketches, 189

Ensuring Safe Food

From Production to Consumption

Executive Summary

Adequate, nutritious, safe food is essential to human survival, but food can also cause or convey risks to health and even life itself. Although estimates vary widely, there is agreement that foodborne illness is a serious problem. In the United States, as many as 81 million illnesses (Archer and Kvenberg, 1985) and up to 9,000 deaths (CAST, 1994) per year have been attributed to food-related hazards. Estimates of the annual cost of medical treatment and lost productivity vary widely, from $6.6 billion to $37.1 billion from seven major foodborne pathogens (Buzby and Roberts, 1997).

The nation's agriculture and food marketing systems have evolved to provide food to a growing and increasingly sophisticated population. Complex processes built on advances in science and technology have been developed to evaluate and manage the risks associated with the changing nature of the food supply. Well-established systems control many food risks, but serious hazards to public health remain.

PURPOSE AND SCOPE OF THE STUDY

As a result of the continuing concern about the food safety system in the United States, Congress commissioned the National Academy of Sciences, through the Agricultural Research Service of the US Department of Agriculture (USDA), to undertake the study that resulted in this report. The charge to the committee was twofold. The committee was asked to (1) assess the effectiveness of the current system to ensure safe food, and (2) provide recommendations on scientific and organizational changes needed to increase the effectiveness of the

1

food safety system. Over a 6 month period, the committee held three meetings as well as two open forums where agency representatives and relevant stakeholders discussed the food safety system. The committee reviewed many documents, including reports on how other countries are reshaping their systems.

This report summarizes the committee's review of food safety in the United States by (1) describing the current US system for food safety and the changing nature of concerns which it encounters, (2) outlining an effective food safety system, (3) identifying the ways in which the current food safety system is inadequate, and (4) providing recommendations to move toward the scientific foundation and organizational structure of a more effective food safety system.

Protecting the safety of food requires attention to a wide range of potential hazards. Food safety is not limited to concerns related to foodborne pathogens, toxicity of chemical substances, or physical hazards, but may also include issues such as nutrition, food quality, labeling, and education. While the scope of this study includes all of these components, this committee's immediate concern focuses on food-related hazards.

1. The Current US Food Safety System

The US food supply is abundant and affordable and is judged by many to present an acceptable level of risk to health. The system has evolved from one that provided consumers with minimally processed basic commodities that were predominantly for home preparation to today's system of highly processed products designed either to be ready-to-eat or to require minimal preparation in the home. As a result of many technological advances, the food system has progressed dramatically from traditional food preservation processes such as salting and curing to today's marketplace with frozen ready-to-eat meals and take-out foods. Likewise, distribution systems for foods have changed greatly.

While these developments have provided the American consumer with a wide array of food products with a high degree of safety, a more diverse food supply carries additional risks as well as benefits. The availability of new food choices such as "minimally processed" vegetable products (for example, prebagged and chopped leaf lettuce mixes) presents new risks for microbial contamination. The globalization of the food system brings food from all parts of the world into the US marketplace, and with it the potential for foodborne infection or other hazards not normally found in the United States.

The current US food safety system has many of the attributes of an effective system. The nature of food safety concerns has changed due to past successful efforts to control the use of unidentified or misrepresented food ingredients and problems with the appearance and wholesomeness of food products; microbiological and chemical hazards now present new and in some cases increasingly serious challenges which cannot be detected using traditional inspection methods. The introduction of Hazard Analysis Critical Control Point (HACCP) monitoring systems in meat, poultry, and seafood products is an example of the introduction of science-based process control methodology into food safety regulation and enforcement.

Many Americans now eat in ways that increase risk, including consuming more raw or minimally processed fruits and vegetables and eating fewer home-prepared meals. A smaller number of food processing and preparation facilities provide food to increasingly larger numbers of US consumers, enhancing the extent of harm that can arise from any one incident. Simultaneously, increasing numbers of Americans have compromised immune systems because of age, illness, or medical treatment. The development of genetically modified foods and modified macronutrients are two examples of new products or technologies that require new ways of evaluating the safety of substances added to the food supply.

The federal government has usually addressed these developments by adding new structures and processes or adjusting old ones. These incremental adjustments have created a number of inefficiencies and apparent conflicts within the system. Some have been addressed (for example, pesticides have been exempted from the Delaney clause's ban on carcinogens), but others remain. USDA is obligated by statute to maintain the system of continuous on-site factory inspection by government inspectors that has been the hallmark of meat and poultry regulation. The Food and Drug Administration (FDA), meanwhile, with a more varied industry to regulate, has relied on selective monitoring, in which far fewer inspectors periodically visit settings where food is produced, processed, or stored to verify compliance with or to uncover violations of its requirements. A result is that in some cases inspectors from these two agencies oversee food processing in the same processing facility at the same time due to the different enabling statutes. Agencies are at times precluded by statute from implementing monitoring or enforcement practices that are based in science.

The size and complexity of the US food system require significant involvement of government at all levels—federal, state, and local; of the food industry—ranging from the producer to food server; of universities; of the news media; and, most importantly, of the consumer, to address adequately the multitude of issues that arise in ensuring safe food. At the federal level, the efforts are currently fragmented, with at least 12 agencies[1] involved in the key functions of safety: monitoring, surveillance, inspection, enforcement, outbreak management, research, and education. Efforts to coordinate federal activities have intensified over the last two years with the National Food Safety Initiative. There are over 50 memoranda of agreement between various agencies related to food safety. The recent proposal to create a Joint Food Safety Research Institute

---

[1]The major federal agencies involved include: the Agricultural Marketing Service, the Animal and Plant Health Inspection Service, the Agricultural Research Service, the Cooperative State Research, Education and Extension Service, the Economic Research Service, the Food Safety and Inspection Service, and the Grain Inspection, Packers and Stockyards Administration of the United States Department of Agriculture; the Centers for Disease Control and Prevention, the Food and Drug Administration, and the National Institutes of Health of the Department of Health and Human Services; the National Marine Fisheries Service of the Department of Commerce; and the Environmental Protection Agency.

between USDA and FDA is an obvious outgrowth of such efforts. Notwithstanding these relatively recent activities, however, there still exist significant barriers to full integration.

Summary Findings: The Current US System for Food Safety

- Has many of the attributes of an effective system;
- is a complex, inter-related activity involving government at all levels, the food industry from farm and sea to table, universities, the media, and the consumer;
- is moving toward a more science-based approach with HACCP and with risk based assessment;
- is limited by statute in implementing practices and enforcement that are based in science;
- is fragmented by having 12 primary federal agencies involved in key functions of safety: monitoring, surveillance, inspection, enforcement, outbreak management, research, and education; and
- is facing tremendous pressures with regard to:
  - emerging pathogens and ability to detect them;
  - maintaining adequate inspection and monitoring of the increasing volume of imported foods, especially fruits and vegetables;
  - maintaining adequate inspection of commercial food services and the increasing number of larger food processing plants; and
  - the growing number of people at high risk for foodborne illnesses.

2. An Effective Food Safety System

Mission

The committee defines safe food as food that is wholesome, that does not exceed an acceptable level of risk associated with pathogenic organisms or chemical and physical hazards, and whose supply is the result of the combined activities of Congress, regulatory agencies, multiple industries, universities, private organizations, and consumers. The mission of a food safety system should be stated as an operational charge that uses and reflects that definition. After reviewing the missions presented by some of the lead federal agencies involved in the US food safety system, the committee defined an overall mission as follows:

> *The mission of an effective food safety system is to protect and improve the public health by ensuring that foods meet science-based safety standards through the integrated activities of the public and private sectors.*

Attributes of an Effective Food Safety System

The attributes of a model food safety system can be summarized in five major components. First, it should be science-based, with a strong emphasis on risk analysis, thus allowing the greatest priority in terms of resources and activity to be placed on the risks deemed to have the greatest potential impact (see Box ES-1). Adjusting effort to risk depends on being able to identify hazards, evaluate the dose-response characteristics of the hazards, estimate or measure exposures, and then determine the likely frequency and severity of effects on health resulting from estimated exposure. Hazards are properties of substances that can cause adverse consequences. Hazards associated with food include microbiological pathogens, naturally occurring toxins, allergens, intentional and unintentional additives, modified food components, agricultural chemicals, environmental contaminants, animal drug residues, and excessive consumption of some dietary supplements. In addition, improper methods of food handling and preparation in the home can contribute to increases in other hazards.

The limited resources available to address food safety issues direct that regulatory priorities be based on risk analysis, which includes evaluation of prevention strategies where possible. This approach enables regulators to estimate the probability that various categories of susceptible persons (for example, the elderly, or nursing mothers) might acquire illness from eating specific foods and thereby allows regulators to place greater emphasis and direct resources on those foods or hazards with the highest risk of causing human illness. Risk analysis provides a science-based approach to address food safety issues. Comprehensive human and animal disease surveillance must be an integral part of any risk analysis in order to estimate exposure.

The second component in a model system is to have a national food law that is clear, rational, and comprehensive, as well as scientifically based on risk. Scientific understanding of risks changes, so federal food safety efforts must be carried out within a flexible framework. US regulatory agencies are moving toward science-based HACCP programs[2]. This is a major step toward a science-based system, but other steps remain critical. An ideal system would be preventive and anticipatory in nature, and thus designed with integrated national surveillance and monitoring along with education and research required to support these activities woven into the fabric of the system. A reliable and accurate system of data collection, processing, evaluation, and transfer is the foundation for scientific risk analysis. Research should have both applied and basic components and be targeted at the needs of producers, processors, consumers, and regulatory decision-makers and other scientists.

---

[2] The implementation of the science-based HACCP strategy is perhaps the most notable recent advance. In contrast to the traditional reactive food safety strategies, the HACCP system focuses on preventing hazards that could cause foodborne illness by applying science-based control processes at each step, from raw material to finished product.

BOX ES-1.   What Is the Meaning of Science-Based?

A science base for ensuring safe food encompasses many elements. When utilized, these elements improve the ability to identify, reduce, and manage risks; minimize occurrence of foodborne hazards; gather and utilize information; enhance knowledge; and improve overall food safety. Several examples of science-based actions that have been implemented in the US food safety system that are readily recognized as positive elements of the system include:

- Implementation of low-acid canned-food processing technology, which reduces the risk of botulism;
- implementation of HACCP systems and risk assessment in decision-making;
- approval of irradiation technology for use in spices, pork, beef, poultry, fruits and vegetables;
- prohibition of the use of lead-based paints on utensils that come in contact with food;
- estimation of maximum allowable exposure levels to pesticides;
- development of standards for allowable practices associated with transport of foods following transport of pesticides in the same containers;
- use of labeling as a device to warn consumers who are sensitive to potential food allergens of the content of the allergen; and
- requirements that meat and poultry products at the retail level carry consumer information related to safe food-handling practices.

While the approaches above are important successful science-based tools in food production and processing, these are only examples of implementation of the scientific basis for food safety. An effective food safety system also integrates science and risk analysis at all levels of the system, including food safety research, information and technology transfer, and consumer education.

Third, a model food safety system should also have a unified mission and a single official who is responsible for food safety at the federal level and who has the authority and the resources to implement science-based policy in all federal activities related to food safety. This would allow for effective and consistent regulation and enforcement. Similar risks require similar planning, action, and response. Thus the intensity, nature, and frequency of inspection should be similar for foods posing similar risks. A central voice is critical to effective marshaling of all aspects of the food safety system to create a coordinated response to foodborne disease outbreaks. Control of resources is also critical in order to encourage movement toward science-based food safety provisions and to ensure that research and education are targeted toward efforts that will produce the greatest benefit for a given cost of improving food safety.

The fourth essential feature of an ideal federal food safety system is that it be organized to be responsive to and work in true partnership with nonfederal partners. These include state and local governments, the food industry, and consumers. The food safety system must function as an integrated enterprise. It must be agile, fluid, connected, integrated, and transparent, with well-defined accountability and responsibility for each partner in the system. It must frame approaches to risk management that recognize the importance of public perception of risks as well as assessments conducted by experts.

Finally, an effective food safety system must be supported by funding adequate to carry out its major functions and mission—to promote the public's health and safety. Moving toward science-based risk analysis as the underpinning of the system should allow reallocation of resources to areas identified as critical to an integrated, focused effort to ensure safe food.

Summary Findings: An Effective Food Safety System

- Should be science-based with a strong emphasis on risk analysis and prevention thus allowing the greatest priority in terms of resources and activity to be placed on the risks deemed to have the greatest potential impact;
- is based on a national food law that is clear, rational, and scientifically based on risk;
- includes comprehensive surveillance and monitoring activities which serve as a basis for risk analysis;
- has one central voice at the federal level which is responsible for food safety and has the authority and resources to implement science-based policy in all federal activities related to food safety;
- recognizes the responsibilities and central role played by the non-federal partners (state, local, industry, consumers) in the food safety system; and
- receives adequate funding to carry out major functions required.

3. Where Current US Food Safety Activities Fall Short

Statutory revision is essential to the development and implementation of an effective and efficient science-based food safety system. Major aspects of the current system are in critical need of attention in order to move toward a more effective food safety system. Food safety in the United States lacks integrated Congressional oversight, allocation of funding based on science, and sustained political support. Statutory impediments interfere with implementation of a more effective food safety system. More than 35 primary statutes regulate food safety. Statutory revision is essential to the development and implementation of an effective and efficient science-based food safety system. The meat and poultry inspection laws mandate a form of compliance monitoring that is largely unrelated to the magnitude or the types of risks that are now posed by those foods. This diverts efforts and perhaps resources from actual risks and other hazards. Inconsistent food statutes often inhibit the use of science-based decision-making in activities related to food safety, including lack of jurisdiction to evaluate food-handling practices in countries of origin for some types of imported foods.

The federal government response to food safety issues is too often crisis-driven. Management decisions, emphasis, and agency culture are driven by the primary concerns of each agency and special initiatives. One result is fragmentation, which causes a lack of coordination and consistency among agencies in mission, food safety policies, regulation, and enforcement. The fact that some agencies have dual responsibilities (regulation of the quality of food products while marketing them via promotional activities) makes their actions more vulnerable to criticism regarding possible conflicts of interest and may bias their approach to food safety.

In addition to fragmented and overlapping authorities, federal activities are not well-integrated with state and local activities. This results in overlapping responsibilities, gaps in responsibilities, and inefficiencies. Although FDA recommended minimum food-handling standards in a Food Code issued in 1993, the Code has not been adopted in its entirety by most state and local authorities. Surveillance efforts currently in place (such as FoodNet) have been designed to provide data representative of national trends with regard to seven indicator foodborne pathogens yet are not designed to identify trends within smaller geographic areas or communities. Similarly, there are conflicts between US requirements and those of other nations and international bodies. These inadequacies have serious implications for both food imports and food exports.

The multi-faceted federal framework of the US food safety system lacks direction from a single leader who can speak for the government when confronting food safety issues and providing answers to the public. There is no single voice in the government to communicate with stakeholders regarding food safety issues. The lack of clear leadership at the federal level impedes the federal role in the management of food safety. Leadership is needed to set priorities, deploy resources, and integrate a consistent policy into all levels of the system.

A significant impediment to moving toward a science-based food safety system is the lack of adequate emphasis on and integration of surveillance activities that provide timely information on current and potential foodborne disease and related hazards. This timely information is critical if the food safety system is to move from a mode of reaction to prevention. FDA's lack of resources to maintain adequate inspection and monitoring of commercial food facilities and of fresh fruits and vegetables, both domestic and imported, using statute-driven methods of monitoring and enforcement, increases the threat of foodborne disease and related hazards in the food supply.

The committee found that the resource base for research and surveillance was not adequate to achieve the goals identified as necessary for an effective system. Furthermore, there is not an adequately coordinated effort on the scale required to analyze risk and respond to the challenges of the changing nature of American food hazards related to increases in consumption of imported foods and of food eaten outside the home.

With respect to consumer education, the committee found two major problems: in some instances, consumer knowledge is inadequate or erroneous; and even where knowledge is adequate, it often fails to influence behavior.

Summary Findings: Where the US Food Safety System Falls Short

- Inconsistent, uneven and at times archaic food statutes that inhibit use of science-based decision-making in activities related to food safety, including imported foods;
- a lack of adequate integration among the 12 primary agencies that are involved in implementing the 35 primary statutes that regulate food safety;
- inadequate integration of federal programs and activities with state and local activities;
- absence of focused leadership: no single federal entity is both responsible for the government's efforts and given the authority to implement policy and designate resources toward food safety activities;
- lack of similar missions with regard to food safety of the various agencies reviewed;
- inadequate emphasis on surveillance necessary to provide timely information on current and potential foodborne hazards;
- resources currently identified for research and surveillance inadequate to support science-based system;
- limited consumer knowledge, which does not appear to have much impact on food-handling behavior; and
- lack of nationwide adherence to appropriate minimum standards.

4. Conclusions and Recommendations Needed to Improve the US Food Safety System

Given the concerns outlined above, the committee came to three primary conclusions:

I. An effective and efficient food safety system must be based in science.

II. To achieve a food safety system based on science, current statutes governing food safety regulation and management must be revised.

III. To implement a science-based system, reorganization of federal food safety efforts is required.

To accomplish these objectives, the committee recommends that the following measures be taken regarding the scientific and organizational changes needed to improve the US food safety system:

Recommendation I:

Base the food safety system on science.

The United States has enjoyed notable successes in improving food safety. One example is the joint government-industry development of low-acid canned food regulations, based on contingency microbiology and food engineering principles, that has almost eliminated botulism resulting from improperly processed commercial food. Similarly, the passage of the 1958 Food Additives Amendment to the Food, Drug, and Cosmetic Act of 1938 was a "technology forcing" event that improved the evaluation of the safety of added and natural substances and reduced the risks associated with the use of food additives. In a like manner, the Delaney clause of that amendment resulted in increased attention to carcinogenic substances in the food supply. With increasing knowledge, many rational, science-based regulatory philosophies have been adopted, some of which rely on quantitative risk assessment. Adoption of such a science-based regulatory philosophy has been uneven and difficult to ensure given the fragmentation of food safety activities, and the differing missions of the various agencies responsible for specific components of food safety. This philosophy must be integrated into all aspects of the food safety system, from federal to state and local.

Recommendation IIa:

Congress should change federal statutes so that inspection, enforcement, and research efforts can be based on scientifically supportable assessments of risks to public health.

Limitations on the resources available to address food safety issues require that food safety activities operate with maximal efficiency within these limits. This does not require full-scale, cost-benefit analysis of each issue, but it does require that costs, risks, and benefits be known with some precision. Thus, where feasible, regulatory priorities should be based on risk analysis which includes evaluation of prevention strategies where possible. The greatest strides in ensuring food safety from production to consumption can be made through a science-based system that ensures that surveillance, regulatory, and research resources are allocated to maximize effectiveness. This will require identification of the greatest public health needs through surveillance and risk analysis, and evaluation of prevention strategies. The state of knowledge and technology defines what is achievable through the application of current science. Public resources can have the greatest favorable effect on public health if they are allocated in accordance with the combined analysis of risk assessment and technical feasibility. However, limiting allocation of resources to *only* those areas where high priority hazards are known can create a significant problem: other hazards with somewhat lower priority but with a much greater probability of reduction or elimination might not be addressed due to limited resources. Thus both the marginal risks and marginal benefits must also be considered in allocating resources.

Not all agencies responsible for monitoring the safety of imported food are authorized to enter into agreements with the governments of exporting countries in order to reciprocally recognize food safety standards or inspection results. Uniform or harmonized food safety standards and practices should be established, and officials allowed to undertake research, monitoring, surveillance, and inspection activities within other countries. This should permit inspection and monitoring efforts to be allocated in accordance with science-based assessments of risk and benefit. Changes in federal statute that would foster and enhance science-based strategies are shown in Box ES-2.

> **BOX ES-2. Changes in Federal Statutes that Would Foster and
>   Enhance Science-based Strategies**
>
> • Eliminate continuous inspection system for meat and poultry and
>   replace with a science-based approach which is capable of
>   detecting hazards of concern;
> • mandate a single set of science-based inspection regulations for all
>   foods; and
> • mandate that all imported foods come from only countries with
>   food safety standards deemed equivalent to US standards.

Recommendation IIb:

> **Congress and the administration should require development of a
> comprehensive national food safety plan. Funds appropriated for
> food safety programs (including research and education programs)
> should be allocated in accordance with science-based assessments
> of risk and potential benefit.**

Changes in statutes or organization should be based on a rational, well-developed national food safety plan formulated by current federal agencies charged with food safety efforts and with representation from the many stakeholders involved in ensuring safe food. Such a plan, as shown in Box ES-3, should serve as the blueprint for strategies designed to determine priorities for funding, to determine what the needs are, and to ensure that they are incorporated into activities and outcome evaluation.

BOX ES-3. The National Food Safety Plan Should

- Include a unified, science-based food safety mission;
- integrate federal, state, and local food safety activities;
- allocate funding for food safety in accordance with science-based assessments of risk and potential benefit;
- provide adequate and identifiable support for the research and surveillance needed to:
  - monitor changes in risk or potential hazards created by changes in food supply or consumption patterns, and
  - improve the capability to predict and avoid new hazards;
- increase monitoring and surveillance efforts to improve knowledge of the incidence, seriousness, and cause-effect relationships of foodborne diseases and related hazards;
- address the additional and distinctive efforts required to ensure the safety of imported foods;
- recognize the burdens imposed on state and local authorities that have primary front-line responsibility for regulation of food service establishments; and
- include a plan to address consumers' behaviors related to safe food-handling practices.

Recommendation IIIa:

> **To implement a science-based system, Congress should establish, by statute, a unified and central framework for managing federal food safety programs, one that is headed by a single official and which has the responsibility and control of resources for all federal food safety activities, including outbreak management, standard-setting, inspection, monitoring, surveillance, risk assessment, enforcement, research, and education.**

The committee was asked to consider organizational changes that would improve the safety of food in the United States. During the 6 months of active review of information and deliberation, the committee identified characteristics needed in an organizational structure that would provide for an improved focus for food safety in the United States. The committee found that the current fragmented regulatory structure is not well-equipped to meet the current challenges. The key recommendation in this regard is that in order for there to be successful structure, one official should be responsible for federal efforts in food safety and have control of resources allocated to food safety.

This recommendation envisions an identifiable, high-ranking, presidentially-appointed head, who would direct and coordinate federal activities and speak to the nation, giving federal food safety efforts a single voice. The structure created, and the person heading it, should have control over the resources Congress allocates to the food safety effort; the structure should also have a firm foundation in statute and thus not be temporary and easily changed by political agendas or executive directives. It is also important that the person heading the structure should be accountable to an official no lower than a cabinet secretary and, ultimately, to the President.

Many members of the committee are of the view that the most viable means of achieving these goals would be to create a single, unified agency headed by a single administrator—an agency that would incorporate the several relevant functions now dispersed, and in many instances separately organized, among three departments and a department-level agency. However, designing the precise structure and assessing the associated costs involved are not possible in the time frame given the committee, nor were they included in its charge. The committee did discuss other possible structures; while it ruled out some, it certainly did not examine all possible configurations and thus the examples provided in Box ES-4 are only illustrative of possible overall structures that could be considered.

BOX ES-4. Some Examples of Possible Organizational Structures to Create a Single Federal Voice for Food Safety

- A Food Safety Council with representatives from the agencies with a central chair appointed by the President, reporting to Congress and having control of resources,

- designating one current agency as the lead agency and having the head of that agency be the responsible individual,

- a single agency reporting to one current cabinet-level secretary, and

- an independent single agency at cabinet level.

NOTE: These examples are provided for illustrative purposes and many other configurations are possible. It is strongly recommended that future activities be directed toward identifying a feasible structure that meets the criteria outlined.

The committee does not believe that the type of centralized focus envisioned can be achieved through appointment of an individual with formal coordinating responsibility but without legal authority or budgetary control for food safety, a model similar to a White House-based 'czar'. Nor, in the committee's view, can this goal be achieved through a coordinating committee similar to that currently provided via the National Food Safety Initiative. In evaluating possible structures, the committee realized that past experience with other structures or reorganizations, including the creation of new agencies, such as the Environmental Protection Agency (EPA), should inform any final judgment. Further, it is quite possible that other models may now exist in government that can serve as templates for structural reform. Whether or not a single agency emerges, the ultimate structure must provide for not just delegated responsibility, but also for control of resources and authority over food safety activities in the federal government.

Recommendation IIIb:

> **Congress should provide the agency responsible for food safety at the federal level with the tools necessary to integrate and unify the efforts of authorities at the state and local levels to enhance food safety.**

This report specifically addresses the federal role in the food safety system, but the roles of state and local government entities are equally critical. For integrated operation of a food safety system, officials at all levels of government must work together in support of common goals of a science-based system. The federal government must be able to ensure nationwide adherence to minimal standards when it is deemed appropriate. The work of the states and localities in support of the federal mission deserves improved formal recognition and appropriate financial support. Statutory tools required to integrate state and local activities regarding food safety into an effective national system are shown in Box ES-5.

BOX ES-5. The Statutory Tools Required to Integrate Local and State Activities Regarding Food Safety into an Effective National System

- Authority to mandate adherence to minimal federal standards for products or processes,

- continued authority to deputize state and local officials to serve as enforcers of federal law,

- funding to support, in whole or in part, activities of state and local officials that are judged necessary or appropriate to enhance the safety of food,

- authority given to the federal official responsible for food safety to direct action by other agencies with assessment and monitoring capabilities, and

- authority to convene working groups, create partnerships, and direct other forms and means of collaboration to achieve integrated protection of the food supply.

MOVING TOWARD A MODEL SYSTEM

It is recognized that these recommendations will need significant review and discussion. The committee focused on the need for a centrally managed federal system to ensure coordination and direction in food safety programs and policy, and to serve as a single voice with authority and resources to suggest and implement legislation. It had insufficient time to review all the possible organizational structures that could accomplish this goal. A successor study could focus on this. Of critical importance, though, are the first two recommendations: the first, to base the system on science, and the second, that of rewriting the current patchwork of federal food statutes that in many cases do not serve to ensure a scientifically supportable and risk-based food safety system, and certainly prevent it from being more cost effective.

Regardless of the organizational structure chosen, a revamped federal food statute is critical to being able to reallocate resources toward risks that have or will have the greatest significance to the public's health. Implementation of these recommendations should not be looked at as a cost-cutting measure, but rather as a way to design a well-defined integrated system to ensure safe food. This system may well be able to demonstrate effectively a need for additional resources to address important and specific problems. Although the National Food Safety Initiative properly seeks to alleviate problems inherent in the present decentralized structure, experience indicates that any ad hoc administrative adjustments and commitments to coordination will not suffice to bring about the vast cultural changes and collaborative efforts needed to create an integrated system.

Changing hazards associated with food and changing degrees of acceptance of risk are factors that impact the nation's ability to protect public health and ensure safe food. Risk acceptance and foodborne hazards will continue to change and evolve with new technologies and consumer demands. Federal food safety efforts must be designed to deal with those changes. This report is not a comprehensive and all-inclusive discussion of these issues. Adoption of the recommendations in this report will not end the effort to make food safer. They should, however, contribute to ensuring the safety of our food while providing a blueprint for a truly integrated system.

1

Introduction and Background

Humans must have food to survive. In the United States and other countries, the system of obtaining food was highly localized before the twentieth century. With the development of new technologies and improved transportation, food production and distribution systems became national in scope and more complex. The current food system stretches from producers to consumers and is international in scope. Ensuring its quantity, nutritional adequacy, and safety has become more complicated, and requires major government and private-sector efforts.

Food safety encompasses a wide spectrum of issues—not only the avoidance of foodborne pathogens, chemical toxicants, and physical hazards, but also issues such as nutrition, food quality, labeling, and education. The system for regulating the food supply in the United States involves all levels of government from federal to local. The present legal framework is comprised of many inconsistent statutes and regulations, and implementing authority is spread among at least 12 federal agencies[1] (Appendix A). Such a fragmented structure requires heroic efforts at cooperation, communication, and coordination (federal agencies have reported more than 50 interagency agreements), but duplication of efforts and regulatory gaps are common. Food safety problems that transcend

---

[1] The major federal agencies involved include: the Agricultural Marketing Service, the Animal and Plant Health Inspection Service, the Agricultural Research Service, the Cooperative State Research, Education and Extension Service, the Economic Research Service, the Food Safety and Inspection Service, and the Grain Inspection, Packers and Stockyards Administration of the United States Department of Agriculture; the Centers for Disease Control and Prevention, the Food and Drug Administration, and the National Institutes of Health of the Department of Health and Human Services; the National Marine Fisheries Service of the Department of Commerce; and the Environmental Protection Agency.

the jurisdictional boundaries of two or more agencies are often not reported in the most expeditious manner. The General Accounting Office (GAO) reports that the National Marine Fisheries Service (NMFS), which operates a voluntary seafood inspection program, failed to notify the Food and Drug Administration (FDA), the agency with regulatory responsibility for corrective action, of 198 plants that failed NMFS inspection between 1988 and 1991 (GAO, 1992).

Recent outbreaks involving such items as Guatemalan raspberries, hamburger, ice cream, and cereal have raised concern over the adequacy of the current system to ensure the safety of the US food supply. The GAO, public interest groups, and several members of Congress have suggested the consolidation of the existing federal food safety structure into a single food safety agency (GAO, 1997). (See Appendix B for a 1998 Congressional Research Service analysis of several proposals.) In addition, the Institute of Food Technologists (IFT) recently developed *Guiding Principles for Optimum Food Safety Oversight and Regulation in the United States*, which describes attributes of an effective food safety system (IFT, 1998). These principles have been endorsed by 13 professional, scientific societies.

To improve the safety of the US food supply, in early 1997 President Clinton directed the Secretary of Agriculture, the Secretary of Health and Human Services, and the Administrator of the Environmental Protection Agency to develop a food safety initiative. *Food Safety from Farm to Table: A National Food-Safety Initiative* (Appendix C) seeks to address hazards that present the greatest risk, make the best use of public and private resources, increase collaboration between public and private organizations, and improve coordination in the government. Recently, President Clinton announced a plan to create a Joint Institute for Food Safety Research that will develop a coordinated strategy for conducting food safety research consistent with the above national initiative (Office of the President, 1998).

CHANGES IN THE US FOOD SYSTEM AND
THEIR EFFECTS ON FOOD SAFETY

The US food supply is abundant and affordable and it is acknowledged by many to pose an acceptable level of risk. The food system has evolved from one that provided consumers with minimally processed basic commodities for home meal preparation to today's availability of highly processed products that are ready-to-eat or require minimal preparation. Food preservation processes have changed dramatically from traditional salting, curing, drying, and heating. Today's products are the result of many technological developments such as pasteurization, irradiation, and genetic engineering. Likewise, food distribution systems have changed greatly. The broad introduction of refrigerated railcars and trucks, freezers, and air transport created a national and now global food system. These changes allow out-of-season availability, convenience, variety, and improved sensory attributes.

The size and complexity of the US food system raise many safety issues, for example:

- The emergence of new foodborne pathogens such as *Escherichia coli* O157:H7 and the re-emergence of previously identified pathogens such as *Salmonella* have resulted in new microbiological hazards.
- Advances in science and technology that allow the development of genetically modified foods and the construction of modified macronutrients require new ways of evaluating the safety of substances added to the food supply, and this need will increase.
- Heightened consumer interest in raw or minimally processed fruits and vegetables, partly in response to dietary recommendations, has created a year-round demand for fresh produce, which can be met out-of-season only through increased imports (GAO, 1998). This increased produce volume requires additional attention to possible contamination of domestic as well as imported fruits and vegetables.
- Americans eat fewer home-prepared meals than ever before, in response to changes in the US workforce and to developments in food processing and food service that offer greater convenience and variety in available foods (FMI, 1998b). The potential for contamination increases as food is handled by more people.
- As technology has advanced, a smaller number of food facilities provide food to larger numbers of US consumers, increasing the extent of harm that can arise from a single incident.
- The remarkable success of modern medicine in extending the lifespan and increasing the quality of life for many people has placed new demands on the food system and on those responsible for guarding its safety. Increasing numbers of people have immune systems that are compromised because of age, illness, or medical treatment. These people are highly susceptible to illness and death from microbial pathogens, and might be more sensitive to new food ingredients and recently identified natural components of the diet.
- Increasing consumption of fortified foods and dietary supplements, including herbals, has raised new questions about the safety of "natural" substances not normally in the diet, or normally part of the diet but at much lower concentrations, and about the health effects of consuming high concentrations of nutrients ordinarily considered safe.

Thus, the developments that have provided the American consumer with a wide array of food products have also introduced risks. Government has attempted to address such developments by adding structures and processes without always considering their effects on other aspects of the system. As a result, inefficiencies and apparent conflicts within the system have arisen. Some have been corrected (for example, pesticides have been exempted from the Delaney clause's ban on carcinogens[2]), but others remain. For example, inspectors from multiple agencies oversee parallel and nearly identical processes in the same food processing facility.

The current food safety system has evolved piecemeal over almost a century in response to changes in the food supply and to changes in the biophysical and social environments in which the system operates. The present system is not the product of planning, and it is often not equipped to anticipate changes. But the situation is not just haphazard; changes in risks have made the system outmoded. The role and organization of government entities have remained largely unchanged, and the food safety system has fallen behind today's needs.

SCOPE OF THE FOOD SAFETY PROBLEM

Over the years, as the agriculture and marketing systems have evolved to provide food to a growing and increasingly sophisticated population, complex processes built on advances in science and technology have been developed to evaluate and manage the risks associated with the food supply. In spite of well-established systems that control many food risks, serious hazards to public health remain. Although estimates vary greatly, there is agreement that foodborne illness is a serious problem. In the United States, an estimated 81 million cases of foodborne illness may occur each year (Archer and Kvenberg, 1985), resulting in as many as 9,000 deaths (CAST, 1994). The estimated annual medical costs and productivity losses due to seven major foodborne pathogens range from $6.6 billion to $37.1 billion (Buzby and Roberts, 1997).

The responsibility for managing foodborne risks is shared throughout the system because the wholesomeness and safety of a food are influenced by all the people and processes that handle or transform it from production to consumption (Sobal et al., in press). Federal, state, and local governments play major roles in managing risks to protect the public from hazards in the food supply. Regulatory agencies are empowered to prescribe rules, standards, and processes to control risks; to develop and maintain research programs to apply contemporary science and technology to safety decisions; to monitor risks in the food supply; and to provide information and education to all components of the food system. In authorizing and funding efforts to ensure the safety of the food supply, the government must balance the interests of diverse groups and allocate finite resources among competing needs.

---

[2] The Delaney clause, which was included in the 1958 Food Additives Amendment to the Food, Drug, and Cosmetics Act, directs that "no additive shall be deemed to be safe if it is found to induce cancer when ingested by man or animal, or if it is found, after tests which are appropriate for the evaluation of the safety of food additives, to induce cancer in man or animal."

Faulty handling of a product at any point in the system can transform a safe product into one that can cause serious harm. Producers, shippers, importers, processors, wholesalers, retailers, handlers, and consumers all influence the health risks associated with food products. Consumers play a particularly important role in the control of microbiological risks, both in their food handling practices and in their demand for an effective, efficient food safety system.

Food safety issues also involve the interplay of domestic and international legal, political, scientific, social, and economic forces. Intense debates about desired levels of protection and about the appropriateness of different control measures can arise as parties discuss the scientific bases for risk decisions, public expectations, and relative costs and benefits of intervention in different ways and in different components of the food system.

Science must play a vital role in food safety decisions through risk assessment, that is, the identification of hazards and the determination of the likelihood and severity of risk under given conditions of exposure (IOM, 1997). Hazards are biological, chemical, or physical substances that can cause adverse consequences. Hazards associated with food include microbiological pathogens, naturally occurring toxins, allergens, intentional and unintentional additives, modified food components, agricultural chemicals, environmental contaminants, animal drug residues, and excessive consumption of some dietary supplements. In addition, certain methods of food preparation in the home can contribute to increasing some of these hazards. However, a hazard does not pose a risk in the absence of exposure. The susceptibility of the consumer and the magnitude of exposure determine whether those hazards cause immunological changes, genetic and developmental changes, cancer, or death.

Hazard identification is the basis for estimating risk. A food safety risk is the probability of harm to health resulting from a food-related hazard at a particular exposure to a specified person or group. It is important to recognize that safety is an intellectual concept, not an inherent biological property of a substance; safety has been defined as the judgment of an acceptable level of risk. Thus, "safe food" involves a subjective evaluation of social issues and values, as well as a scientific assessment of risk (Lowrance, 1976; Miller, 1997).

HISTORY OF US FOOD SAFETY REGULATION

In the United States, regulation of food safety was largely the responsibility of state and local officials until the first decade of the twentieth century. Nineteenth century legal theorists questioned whether the US Constitution gave Congress the authority to legislate matters of health and safety. The emergence of a national market for food, combined with shocking stories of practices in the food industry, spurred the federal government to reassess its responsibility to ensure food safety. In response, in 1906 Congress passed the Meat Inspection

Act and the Pure Food and Drugs Act, the first national laws designed to protect consumers against foodborne illness.

Although those seminal laws provide the basic legal and institutional framework for the federal regulation of food safety that we observe today, they are very different in their implementation and responsibilities. Their core was similar: each prohibited the shipment in interstate commerce of food that met any of several definitions of "adulteration." Those definitions, or proscriptions, targeted products that were spoiled, contaminated with filth, derived from diseased animals, or contained unsafe substances. In short, both laws sought to prevent the sale of food that could offend consumers or cause them to become ill.

The original Meat Inspection Act and Pure Food and Drugs Act focused on different sectors of the food market and, from the beginning, supported different approaches to ensuring compliance. The Meat Inspection Act, which has been administered by the US Department of Agriculture (USDA) since its inception, requires continuous on-site factory inspections by government inspectors using sight, smell, and touch to detect problems. The USDA also administers the 1957 Poultry Products Inspection Act, which requires continuous inspection of poultry and poultry products and the 1970 Egg Product Inspection Act, which requires continuous inspection of the processing of liquid, frozen, and dried egg products. Animal carcasses and processed products cannot be shipped from the processing plant until they have been inspected and deemed to be unadulterated by the USDA inspector.

The 1906 Pure Food and Drugs Act was administered by the USDA Bureau of Chemistry, which was renamed the Food and Drug Administration (FDA) in 1930. In 1940, FDA was transferred to the Federal Security Agency, and in 1953 it became a separate entity in the Department of Health, Education, and Welfare, later retitled the Department of Health and Human Services. FDA, with a more varied and ever-expanding industry to regulate, has used a sampling strategy in which far fewer inspectors pay periodic visits to settings where food is produced, processed, or stored to verify compliance with its requirements or to uncover and punish violations. In 1958, when Congress enacted the Food Additives Amendment to the Food, Drug, and Cosmetic Act of 1938, the FDA was given premarket review and approval authority over chemical additives to foods.

The meat and poultry inspection system still requires sight, smell, and touch inspections, which are ineffective in addressing the current issues of food safety. Expert opinion that USDA inspection procedures do not adequately address the microbiological problems associated with meat and poultry (NAS, 1987; 1990) led to the adoption of a new approach to inspection using the Hazard Analysis Critical Control Point (HACCP) system (NAS, 1985). In contrast to the reactive characteristics of traditional food safety strategies, the HACCP system focuses on preventing hazards that could cause foodborne illness by applying science-based controls at each step of the process from raw material to finished product.

Following the recommendation of a National Academy of Sciences committee, FDA adopted the HACCP approach for seafood inspection in December 1995, and USDA began the implementation of HACCP for meat and poultry inspection in January 1997 with completion of the implementation by January 2000 (FDA, 1995; FSIS, 1996b, 1998).

Agencies other than USDA and FDA—such as the National Marine Fisheries Service (NMFS) in the Department of Commerce, the Environmental Protection Agency (EPA), the Centers for Disease Control and Prevention (CDC), and the National Institutes of Health (NIH)—also have roles in food safety. NMFS conducts a voluntary seafood inspection and grading program and does research on seafood safety. The EPA Office of Prevention, Pesticides, and Toxic Substances is responsible for risk assessment, product approvals, tolerance setting, and research on pesticide residues in or on human food and animal feed. State health departments in conjunction with CDC are responsible for the surveillance and investigation of illnesses related to foods, and NIH conducts research related to foodborne disease. Many state and local agencies are also involved in food safety regulation and inspection.

With so many agencies involved in food safety, decisions and priorities often focus on specific issues rather than strategies, and they are not always well-integrated. The system that has evolved in the federal government for regulating food safety is complex, fragmented, and cumbersome.

THE COMMITTEE AND ITS CHARGE

Congress (HR 2160 Conference Report) directed USDA's Agricultural Research Service to contract with the National Academy of Sciences to conduct a study on the scientific and organizational needs of an effective food safety system. The Academy appointed an ad hoc Food Safety Oversight Commission composed of selected members of the Institute of Medicine's Food and Nutrition Board, the National Research Council's (NRC) Board on Agriculture, and the NRC Commission on Life Science's Board on Environmental Studies and Toxicology; in turn, the ad hoc commission convened the Committee to Ensure Safe Food from Production to Consumption.

The committee was charged with determining the scientific basis of an effective food safety system; assessing the effectiveness of the current US system to ensure safe food; identifying scientific and organizational needs and gaps in the current system at the federal level; and providing recommendations to move toward the scientific foundation and organizational structure of a more effective food safety system for present and future generations. If organizational changes were recommended, a subsequent study on implementing the recommendations was to follow, if requested. Given the constraints on time and funding, the committee focused on the role of the federal government in ensuring safe food.

The committee is aware that safe food is and always will be a moving target with respect to both changing hazards and changing degrees of acceptance of risk. This report is not and cannot be a comprehensive, all-inclusive discussion of these issues and adoption of its recommendations will not end the effort to make food safer. It is not possible to foresee how risk acceptance will change or how the problems will change in decades to come, but federal food safety efforts must be designed effectively to deal with what is known and what is not known.

2

The Current US Food Safety System

Every organization and every person involved with the food chain from farm and sea to table shares responsibility for the safety of food. Our "food safety system" includes producers, processors, shippers, retailers, food preparers, and, ultimately, consumers. The government plays an important role by establishing standards and overseeing their enforcement. Supporting roles are played by trade and consumer organizations that inform policy and by professional organizations and academic institutions that engage in research and education. Great responsibility lies with consumers who must be cognizant of the level of safety associated with the foods they purchase and who must handle these foods accordingly. The food safety system in this country is complex and multilevel. It is also essentially uncoordinated. As a consequence, the government's role is also complex, fragmented, and in many ways uncoordinated.

The committee heard testimony from diverse groups asserting that the US food supply is among the safest in the world (Appendix D), yet found little evidence to either support or contradict this assertion. In fact, surveillance and reporting systems are insufficient in scope, resources, and statutory authority to generate reliable current measures of foodborne illness, much less to establish trends.

This chapter describes the main features of the current food safety system, including regulation, surveillance, research and development, consumer education, and international dimensions. This overview does not provide a detailed description of the system, but it does illustrate where current responsibilities and allocations of resources exist and how the system currently functions.

REGULATION

Federal Regulatory Programs

At least a dozen federal agencies implementing more than 35 statutes make up the federal part of the food safety system. Twenty-eight House and Senate committees provide oversight of these statutes. The primary Congressional committees responsible for food safety are the Agriculture Committee and Commerce Committee in the House; the Agriculture, Nutrition, and Forestry Committee and the Labor and Human Resources Committee in the Senate; and the House and Senate Agriculture, Rural Development, and Related Agencies Appropriating Subcommittees.

Four agencies play major roles in carrying out food safety regulatory activities: the Food and Drug Administration (FDA), which is part of the Department of Health and Human Services (DHHS); the Food Safety and Inspection Service (FSIS) of the US Department of Agriculture (USDA); the Environmental Protection Agency (EPA); and the National Marine Fisheries Service (NMFS) of the Department of Commerce. More than 50 interagency agreements have been developed to tie the activities of the various agencies together.

FDA has jurisdiction over domestic and imported foods that are marketed in interstate commerce, except for meat and poultry products. FDA's Center for Food Safety and Applied Nutrition (CFSAN) seeks to ensure that these foods are safe, sanitary, nutritious, wholesome, and honestly and adequately labeled. CFSAN exercises jurisdiction over food processing plants and has responsibility for approval and surveillance of food-animal drugs, feed additives and of all food additives (including coloring agents, preservatives, food packaging, sanitizers, and boiler water additives) that can become part of food. CFSAN enforces tolerances for pesticide residues that are set by EPA and shares with FSIS responsibilities for egg products (FDA, personal communication to committee, March 1998). The FDA's statutes give CFSAN jurisdiction over restaurants, but it has always ceded this responsibility to states and localities. The agency provides leadership for state regulation of retail and institutional food service through the development of a model Food Code, which it recommends be adopted by states and localities (DHHS, 1995; 1997a).

FDA has oversight responsibility for an estimated 53,000 domestic food establishments (Rawson and Vogt, 1998). In fiscal year 1997, FDA devoted 2,728 staff-years to food safety activities (Lisa Siegel, FDA, personal communication to committee, July 1998). Food safety consumes about 23.5 percent of FDA's budget each year (OMB, 1998). In 1997, that amounted to approximately $203 million for food safety surveillance, risk assessment, research, inspection, and education out of the total FDA budget of $997 million (Appendix E; Lisa Siegel, FDA, personal communication to committee, July 1998). The largest share of FDA's budget is devoted to its nonfood responsibilities including drugs, cosmetics, and medical devices. The agency's culture and its public image have been dominated by its drug approval mission.

FSIS seeks to ensure that meat and poultry products for human consumption are safe, wholesome, and correctly marked, labeled, and packaged if they move into interstate or international commerce. By the mid-1990s, roughly 7,400 FSIS inspectors were responsible for inspecting 6,200 meat and poultry slaughtering and processing plants by continuous carcass-by-carcass inspection during slaughter as well as by full daily inspection during processing (FSIS, 1996b). FSIS shares responsibility with FDA for the safety of intact-shell eggs and processed egg products. Because of the statutorily mandated continuous inspection requirements, FSIS's inspection budget is about four times that of FDA (Appendix E; Thomas Billy, FSIS, personal communication to committee, March 1998). Food scientists believe that inspection of each animal carcass is no longer the best or most cost-effective means of preventing foodborne diseases, but this effort is required by statute and so is fully funded. The sensory evaluation inspection methods used in FSIS inspections were appropriate when adopted 70 years ago, when major concerns included gross contamination, evidence of animal disease, and other problems that are no longer acute concerns. Those methods are not appropriate or adequate to detect the major microbial and chemical hazards of current concern.

Because of the FDA-USDA jurisdictional split along commodity lines, some food products that might be perceived by consumers as similar are regulated differently, depending on content. The most cited example is pizza, which is regulated by FDA unless topped with 2 percent or more of cooked meat or poultry, in which case it is USDA-regulated (FSIS, 1996a; 9 CFR 319.600). This means that inspection at pizza production facilities must be conducted simultaneously under two sets of guidelines by two different inspectors from separate agencies.

EPA licenses all pesticide products distributed in the United States and establishes tolerances for pesticide residues in or on food commodities and animal feed. EPA is responsible for the safe use of pesticides, as well as food-plant detergents and sanitizers, to protect people who work with and around them and to protect the general public from exposure through air, water, and home and garden applications, as well as food uses. EPA is also responsible for protecting against other environmental chemical and microbial contaminants in air and water that might threaten the safety of the food supply (EPA, personal communication to committee, May 1998). In both programs, EPA works with state and local officials.

NMFS conducts a voluntary seafood inspection and grading program which is primarily a food quality activity. Seafood is the only major food source that is both "caught in the wild" and raised domestically. Seafood is an international commodity for which quality and safety standards vary widely from country to country. Inspection of processing is a challenge because much of it takes place at sea (NMFS, personal communication to committee, March 1998). Mandatory regulation of seafood processing is under FDA, and applies to all seafood related entities in FDA's establishment inventory, including exporters, all foreign processors that export to the United States, and importers. However, fishing vessels, common carriers, and retail establishments are excluded.

The Agricultural Marketing Service (AMS), Grain Inspection, Packers, and Stockyards Administration (GIPSA), and Animal and Plant Health Inspection Service (APHIS) of the USDA oversee the USDA's marketing and regulatory programs. Together they play indirect roles in food safety and more direct roles in marketing, surveillance, data collection, and quality assurance (USDA, personal communication to committee, May 1998).

The Centers for Disease Control and Prevention (CDC) of DHHS engages in surveillance and investigation of illnesses associated with food consumption in support of the USDA and FDA regulatory missions (Morris Potter, CDC, personal communication to committee, March 1998). The Federal Trade Commission, through regulation of food advertising, plays an indirect role in food safety regulation.

Several other federal agencies have smaller but important regulatory responsibilities in food safety. For example, the Department of the Treasury's Bureau of Alcohol, Tobacco, and Firearms is responsible for overseeing the production, distribution, and labeling of alcoholic beverages, except for wines containing less than 7 percent alcohol, which are the responsibility of FDA. The department's Customs Service assists other agencies in ensuring the safety and quality of imported foods through such services as collecting samples.

State and Local Regulatory Systems

State and local health departments are responsible for surveillance at the state and local level and the extent to which these activities are carried out varies widely by jurisdiction. States and territories have separate departments of health and of agriculture. In addition, many counties and many cities have parallel agencies. In total, more than 3,000 state and local agencies have food safety responsibilities for retail food establishments (DHHS, 1997a). In many jurisdictions, there is a split between agriculture and health department authority that mirrors, in many respects, the split in federal food safety jurisdictions. In most state and local jurisdictions, for example, the health department has authority over restaurants, but the agriculture department has authority over supermarkets. Thus, a restaurant in a supermarket might be under agriculture department authority, whereas a stand-alone restaurant in the same chain will fall under the authority of the health department. Like FDA and USDA, health and agriculture departments in the same jurisdiction are generally governed by different statutes, use different methods and standards, and have different cultures that affect their regulatory stance.

States are responsible for the inspection of meat and poultry sold in the state where they are produced, but FSIS monitors the process. The 1967 Wholesome Meat Act and the 1968 Wholesome Poultry Products Act require state inspection programs to be "at least equal to" the federal inspection programs. If a state chooses to end its inspection programs or cannot maintain the "at least equal to" standard, FSIS must assume responsibility for inspection. In a few states, state employees carry out inspections in some federal plants under federal-state cooperative inspection agreements.

FDA's Food Code provides scientific standards and guidelines that states and localities may adopt for food safety in restaurants and institutional food settings (DHHS, 1995; 1997a). The code includes temperature standards for cooking, cooling, refrigerating, reheating, and holding food. It also recommends that inspectors visit restaurants every six months. Each state or locality may choose to adopt any or all of the code in its laws or regulations. Although there appears to be some recent progress toward more widespread adoption of this model code (FDA, personal communication to committee, June 1998), there is much variation among jurisdictions in standards currently being applied to restaurants and other food establishments, according to one recent survey (DeWaal and Dahl, 1997).

In contrast with the FDA Food Code, which has had varied acceptance, the Public Health Service 1924 Standard Milk Ordinance has been adopted by all 50 states, the District of Columbia, and US trust territories. This model was created collaboratively by public and private entities to assist states and municipalities in initiating and maintaining effective programs for the prevention of milkborne disease. Now known as the Grade A Pasteurized Milk Ordinance, it is the standard used in the voluntary cooperative state-PHS program for certification of interstate milk shippers. Revisions are considered every two years on the basis of recommendations of the National Conference on Interstate Milk Shipments. The ordinance is incorporated by reference into federal specifications for procurement of milk and milk products, and it is used as the sanitary regulation for milk and milk products served on interstate carriers. The ordinance is recognized by public health agencies, the milk industry, and many others as a national standard for milk sanitation, although exemptions allow for the sale of raw milk in some states (International Dairy Foods Association, personal communication to committee, April 1998).

HACCP Systems

Many parts of the current food safety assurance system are in the early stages of transition to Hazard Analysis Critical Control Point (HACCP) programs. The leadership of FSIS, FDA, and industry in making this fundamental change to a hazard prevention system is commendable. It is widely accepted by the scientific community that use of HACCP systems in food production, processing, distribution, and preparation is the best known approach to enhancing the safety of foods. If HACCP programs are fully implemented, they will substantially increase the effectiveness of the system. HACCP programs use a systematic approach to identify microbiological, chemical, and physical hazards in the food supply, and establish critical control points that eliminate or control such hazards (NRC, 1985). The control must effectively address the identified hazard and the effectiveness of the control point must be validated.

This approach appears to be much more effective in ensuring the safety of foods than traditional visual inspection practices. The HACCP system institutes methods to control food safety hazards, whereas traditional inspection and testing procedures are not designed to detect and control contaminants that are sporadically distributed throughout foods and are not visible.

In 1995, the FDA issued its final rule on HACCP for seafood, requiring all seafood processors to conduct a hazard analysis to determine whether food safety hazards are reasonably likely to occur (FDA, 1995). If no hazards are identified, no HACCP plan is needed, but reassessments are required whenever procedures are changed significantly. Written HACCP plans for seafood must be specific to each location and type of seafood product. In response to the need to train members of the seafood industry in HACCP techniques, the National Seafood HACCP Alliance for Training and Education was created. This organization provides information on HACCP training courses, as well as sample HACCP models for various seafood products.

The Pathogen Reduction and HACCP system regulation of USDA establishes requirements in an effort to reduce the occurrence and numbers of pathogens on meat and poultry products and reduce the incidence of foodborne illness associated with consuming these products. Regulatory performance standards for pathogen reduction and end-product testing to determine whether the HACCP system meets those standards are basic to the USDA's approach to HACCP.

In January 1998, 312 large (over 500 employees) meat and poultry processing plants were required by FSIS to implement HACCP systems. About 6,100 medium and small (10 to 500 employees) processing plants will be required to implement HACCP systems within two years (FSIS, 1996b; FSIS, 1997; FSIS 1998). During the first three months of implementation of HACCP-based inspection by large meat and poultry processors, enforcement actions against 13 plants were taken by FSIS to address system failures and improper implementation or misunderstanding of HACCP procedures by processors or inspectors (FSIS, 1998). In response to the need to train members of the meat and poultry industry, the international meat and poultry HACCP alliance was formed at Texas A&M University. The alliance is composed of industry associations and is affiliated with federal agencies, universities, and professional organizations.

Implementation of HACCP is the responsibility of food producers, processors, distributors, and consumers. The role of government is to ensure that HACCP programs are properly implemented throughout the food supply continuum by evaluation of HACCP plans and inspection of records indicating monitoring of critical control points. Implementation of this innovative approach requires a major educational effort and cultural change among federal inspectors. Adequate resources have not been provided to enable the implementation of HACCP-based inspection effectively, efficiently, and without disruption.

Voluntary Efforts

Trade Associations

Trade associations are formed, in part, to give members a unified voice on various issues of common interest, such as marketing, technical issues, and regulation. Trade associations have been established at the national, state, and regional levels for the following:

- *Food producers.* Examples include the United Fresh Fruit and Vegetable Association, the National Pork Producers Council (NPPC), the National Cattlemen's Beef Association (NCBA), the Animal Health Institute, and the United Egg Producers.
- *Food processors.* Examples include the National Food Processors Association (NFPA), the Grocery Manufacturers of America (GMA), the National Fisheries Institute, the American Meat Institute (AMI), and the International Dairy Foods Association.
- *Food ingredient suppliers.* Examples include the International Food Additive Council and the Sugar Association.
- *Food retailers.* An example is the Food Marketing Institute (FMI).
- *Food service establishments.* Examples include the National Restaurant Association (NRA) and the American School Food Service Association.

Many trade associations have model policies and regulatory support programs to help members enhance food safety and meet regulatory requirements. The NFPA has developed model manuals on managing food product recalls, threats of tampering, and other crises; the manuals can be adapted to a company's needs. Videos and individual training programs are also available to members. The NFPA laboratories historically have helped members and FDA work out questions on the safety of canned and other processed foods (Rhona Applebaum, NFPA, personal communication to committee, April 1998). An industry initiative in the early 1970s led to the low-acid canned foods regulations.

Consumer Groups

Consumer organizations play important roles in the promotion of food safety, including its regulatory aspects. Some of these organizations—such as Consumers Union, the Consumer Federation of America, and the National Consumers League—were formed for general consumer protection purposes. Others—such as the Center for Science in the Public Interest (CSPI), Safe Tables Our Priority, and Public Voice for Food and Health Policy—coalesced primarily around issues of food safety and quality. As opinion leaders, these groups focus public attention on issues of concern, often seeking improved regulatory efforts and outcomes. Some of them, most notably Consumers Union and CSPI, have the scientific, financial, and public information resources to engage in product testing and surveillance and to disseminate their test results. For example, a story about the microbiological safety of poultry, published by Consumers Union in *Consumer Reports* in March 1998, received wide media coverage and effectively focused public attention on food safety concerns.

Professional Organizations

Professional organizations offer expertise to assist both research and regulatory processes. Because members are typically professionals working in all areas of a discipline (industry, government, and academe), these organizations also can offer a more balanced view of issues than might be obtained from experts in any one sector alone. Examples of these organizations include the Institute of Food Technologists (IFT); the American Society for Microbiology; the International Association of Milk, Food, and Environmental Sanitarians; and the Association of Food and Drug Officials. These organizations deliberate and comment on proposals concerning food safety technical and regulatory issues, develop and publish model codes, provide training to industry, sponsor symposia and seminars at annual meetings, publish authoritative technical journals (for example, *Food Technology* and the *Journal of Food Protection*), and publish valuable reference books. A recent example is a document that IFT submitted to the committee, *Guiding Principles for Optimum Food Safety Oversight and Regulation in the United States* (IFT, 1998).

Academe

Universities are actively involved in the food safety system in many ways. Training and continuing education for professionals are key roles played by academe. Specifically designed courses educate inspectors in the health hazards associated with foods, in inspection procedures for identifying foodborne hazards, and in methods used to eliminate these hazards. These programs have been conducted at Texas A&M University for FSIS inspectors and at several other cooperating universities for FDA inspectors. Universities also train state and local regulatory professionals and provide periodic programs on food safety to update producers, processors, retailers, nutritionists, and health professionals. Through outreach and public information programs, universities help the mass media and consumers understand and act on food safety concerns. FDA has cooperative research programs at the Joint Institute for Food Safety and Applied Nutrition at the University of Maryland and at the National Center for Food Safety and Technology at the Illinois Institute of Technology. These programs provide research data necessary to support changes in food safety regulations. For example, proper risk assessment for exposure to a mycotoxin requires knowledge about the stability of mycotoxins during food processing. Recycling is generally to be encouraged, but research on food packaging made from recycled materials would first be necessary to determine the safety of such practices, because nonfood products might have migrated into the recycled materials.

Liability

Failures of food safety can be costly for the food industry. Injured consumers might recover compensation if they are able to trace their illness to a particular food (which is not always possible). In most states, injured consumers benefit from the doctrine of strict product liability and do not have to prove any fault on the part of the producer or distributor if a food causes harm. Indeed, tainted food cases were largely responsible for the development and expansion of strict liability doctrine. Although the doctrine of strict liability (or recovery without proof of fault on the part of the seller) is controversial in some contexts, it has not elicited any substantial outcry with respect to food-related harms.

Because it might be difficult to show that one's illness was in fact food related and to trace it to a particular product, the risk of having to pay damages to consumers for harm is probably not a major incentive for food safety. However, sellers of food that is, or is said to be unsafe, face huge public relations risks, which often prove to be more effective in "regulating" industry. The public is quick to shun whole categories of food products alleged to be tainted, as sellers of cranberries (the pesticide scare of 1959), apples (the Alar scare in 1989), and strawberries (the California Cyclospora scare, which turned out to be caused by raspberries, of 1996), verify. Because many unprocessed food commodities do not carry brand names, a food safety failure can harm careful as well as careless producers. Brand name food producers recognize that a recall or problem with any of their products will have a negative effect throughout their product lines. Most large food companies therefore try to work with suppliers and retailers to ensure that their products are kept safe beyond their immediate premises; the brand name is what the consumer sees.

SURVEILLANCE

Human and Animal Disease

Surveillance for human foodborne diseases is primarily the responsibility of state and local health departments, which are required or authorized to collect and investigate reports of communicable diseases. Although specific reporting requirements vary by state, such common and serious bacterial foodborne pathogens as *Salmonella, Shigella, Campylobacter*, and *E. coli* O157:H7 are reportable in most states. In addition, recognized outbreaks of foodborne disease are reportable in most states regardless of cause. Investigations are conducted to identify cases of illness, determine their sources, and control outbreaks. Responsibility for the primary investigation of individual cases or outbreaks may lie with local and state health departments. This system results in regional disparities in the probability of detecting outbreaks and may affect the thoroughness of an investigation.

On a national level, the CDC collects data from the states on the occurrence of specific pathogens such as *Salmonella, Shigella, Campylobacter*, and *E. coli*, and collects summary data on foodborne disease outbreaks investigated by local and state health departments. CDC conducts field investigations of foodborne diseases only at the request of state health departments. CDC also plays a role in coordinating investigations of multistate or international outbreaks. The FDA and FSIS are called into investigations when the safety of a food in their jurisdictions is questioned. The FDA and FSIS are charged with ensuring that foods implicated in a foodborne illness outbreak and traveling in interstate commerce are removed from the market. Most recalls of food products regulated by FDA and FSIS, whether requested by the agency or initiated by the private entity, are carried out voluntarily by the businesses that manufacture, distribute, or sell these products. By statute they must use different methods to achieve that charge; FSIS uses its recall authority and FDA requests voluntary recalls of hazardous food by industry.

The *Food Safety from Farm to Table: National Food-Safety Initiative* (Appendix C) includes plans to develop elements of an improved foodborne-disease surveillance system. Although it is intended to eventually provide a "new early warning system for foodborne disease surveillance," it takes only the first steps toward such a system. The first component of the system is the Active Foodborne Disease Surveillance System, known as FoodNet. This is a collaborative effort among the CDC, FDA, USDA, and states participating in CDC's Emerging Infections Program. FoodNet is designed to conduct population-based active surveillance of seven bacterial foodborne pathogens (*Salmonella, Shigella, Campylobacter, E. coli* O157: H7, *Listeria, Yersinia*, and *Vibrio*) and determine—through a series of surveys of laboratories, physicians, and the population—the magnitude of diarrheal illnesses and the proportion of these illnesses that are attributable to foods. FoodNet provides one model for studying emerging infections; however, its current focus is limited to these seven routinely identifiable pathogens (Appendix C).

A second major activity of the National Food Safety Initiative is the National Molecular Surveillance Network, or PulseNet, established by CDC in collaboration with state laboratories of public health. In 1996, standard protocols for subtyping *E. coli* O157:H7 with pulsed-field gel electrophoresis (PFGE) were developed to more accurately identify routes of pathogen transmission. PFGE technology allows public health laboratories in different regions of the United States to share information through a national computer network. Epidemiologists can now trace and detect foodborne pathogens up to five times faster than previous surveillance methods (DHHS, 1998).

FSIS surveillance activities include monitoring programs for *Listeria monocytogenes* in cooked and ready-to-eat meat and poultry products; *E. coli* O157:H7 in raw ground beef products, imported products, and food in retail establishments; and *Salmonella* in egg products.

In addition, FSIS conducts "swab tests on premises" to detect antibiotics in meat and poultry and "calf antibiotic and sulfa tests." These systems are being replaced with a new surveillance tool, the "fast antimicrobial-screen test." The FSIS also operates a nationwide "residue violation information system" to check for drug, pesticide, and other chemical residues in slaughtered livestock and poultry and in processed eggs.

FDA's Center for Veterinary Medicine has a new monitoring system to determine trends in antimicrobial resistance and changes in susceptibility. Samples from diagnostic laboratories, slaughter plants, farms, and public health settings are taken and compared for relative differences (Stephen Sundlof, Center for Veterinary Medicine, FDA, personal communication to committee, March 1998).

The National Animal Health Monitoring System (NAHMS) program, under the auspices of APHIS, is designed to serve as a comprehensive system to measure the incidence of and determine the trends in and economic burden of diseases in food producing animals on local, state, and national bases. The NAHMS is administered by the Center for Epidemiology and Animal Health and is closely associated with surveys and data from food animal commodity groups and state departments of agriculture.

USDA requires that certain animal diseases be reported, and each state also has its own listing of reportable diseases. USDA operates a national diagnostic laboratory reference center in two locations—the National Veterinary Services Laboratory in Ames, Iowa, and the Foreign Animal Disease Diagnostic Laboratory at Plum Island, New York. These centers monitor disease-eradication programs, some imported animal products, and reported occurrences of animal diseases across the country. A national infrastructure of animal health diagnostic laboratories across the country, associated with colleges of veterinary medicine or state departments of agriculture, provides an additional avenue for animal disease surveillance that is not federally mandated. These laboratories are excellent sources of information for identifying disease trends and new emerging disease conditions.

Chemical Residues and Environmental Contaminants

Responsibility for monitoring chemical residues and environmental contaminants in food is dispersed among many agencies; primary responsibility rests with FDA and several agencies in USDA, EPA, and NMFS. Frequently, one agency might be responsible for approving a chemical's use, while another is responsible for monitoring residues of that chemical in the food supply. For example, EPA is responsible for approving uses of pesticides on food crops and for setting tolerances, but the testing of foods for pesticide residues is the responsibility of USDA (for meat, poultry, and egg products) and FDA (for all other foods). Brief descriptions of agency programs follow; details can be found elsewhere (GAO, 1994b).

Food and Drug Administration

FDA implements the Federal Food Drug and Cosmetic Act by monitoring foods to ensure that approved chemicals and environmental contaminants are within permissible levels. A wide variety of raw agricultural commodities, processed foods, and animal feeds are tested for pesticide residues, environmental contaminants (such as mycotoxins and heavy metals), industrial chemicals, animal drugs, and other potential contaminants.

US Department of Agriculture

The FSIS is responsible for monitoring meat, poultry, and eggs for pesticides, animal drugs, and environmental contaminants.

The AMS has responsibility to maintain standards for shell egg surveillance and to ensure the proper disposal of restricted eggs, which are shell eggs that may be dirty, cracked, leaking, or otherwise unsuitable for consumer purchase.

The GIPSA's Federal Grain Inspection Service provides federal quality and safety standards and a system for applying them to US grain for both domestic consumption and export.

The National Agricultural Statistics Service (NASS), in conjunction with AMS, monitors chemical residues in foods via the Pesticide Data Program. The AMS collects data on pesticide levels as measured in fruits and vegetables, whereas NASS collects data from farmers about pesticide use on fruits, vegetables, nuts, and field crops.

Environmental Protection Agency

As noted above, EPA registers pesticides and pesticide excipients for use in the United States and establishes tolerances for food and feeds. Enforcement of tolerances is the responsibility of other agencies (FDA or FSIS). Therefore, EPA monitoring of pesticides and industrial chemicals in food is a limited part of its monitoring of these contaminants in the environment.

EPA is responsible for establishing criteria to be used by the states to develop water quality standards. Under the Clean Water Act, EPA has the authority to set standards to restore or maintain the integrity of the nation's waters, which directly affect the safety of fish, shellfish, and wildlife (as well as water for human consumption). EPA is also responsible for enforcing standards for drinking water set under the Safe Drinking Water Act. Water for food processing must be safe and potable as defined by these standards. (FDA regulates bottled water under separate regulations, although there are many cross-references to EPA regulations.)

National Marine Fisheries Service

NMFS conducts a voluntary inspection of seafood processing plants, fishing vessels, and seafood products. FDA has regulatory responsibility for ensuring seafood safety, and NMFS coordinates its inspection efforts with FDA's Office of Seafood Safety. FDA, working with the seafood industry, adopted a mandatory HACCP program for seafood in late 1995 (FDA, 1995).

Federal-State Cooperative Agreements

Many federal monitoring programs rely on cooperation with state agencies for some aspects of administration. For example, FDA has a memorandum of understanding with the National Conference on Interstate Milk Shipments, a voluntary organization of state officials, under which the states carry out much of the monitoring and enforcement to oversee the safety and wholesomeness of fresh milk and cream. A part of this responsibility is testing milk and cream for food animal drug residues. Some of FDA's contracts with the states cover programs to monitor pesticide residues in foods, drug residues in edible animal tissue, and toxins in shellfish.

Industry

The food producing and processing industries conduct substantial chemical surveillance as part of their own safety, quality, and regulatory compliance programs. Their focus is typically on pesticide residues, residues of veterinary drugs, mycotoxins, heavy metals, chemical contaminants, and bacterial pathogens that might be associated with foods. The extent and consistency of these programs are difficult to assess because the data are largely unavailable, except for a few databases maintained through trade associations. Although these programs play an important role in ensuring food safety, the best opportunity to establish an integrated monitoring system lies in the public sector, with oversight provided under regulatory authority. To that end, there might be opportunities for industry and agencies to share information more effectively.

TECHNICAL GUIDANCE AND EDUCATION

Government Activities

An array of government programs offers technical guidance and education on producing and processing safe foods. NMFS has developed one of the few federal programs to provide food safety technical guidance at the producer level. Meat, poultry, dairy, egg, produce, grain, and legume producers receive little or no federal technical assistance on food safety issues. FSIS inspectors and administrators are available to address food safety issues related to meat, poultry, and egg processing, while AMS certifiers provide processors of fresh cut produce advice on a "qualified through verification" program that includes implementation of HACCP plans. The FDA provides technical guidance on HACCP-related matters to processors of foods other than meat, poultry, and eggs.

Several federal programs provide consumer education on food safety issues. The USDA consumer hotline responds to thousands of consumer inquiries a year about food safety and prepares and distributes food safety tips for consumers. CDC, often in collaboration with FDA and USDA, prepares videos and brochures about safe food preparation and consumption by high-risk populations, such as people who are immunocompromised, pregnant, or elderly. A recently introduced "Fight BAC" program, jointly sponsored by USDA, DHHS, and the food industry, is a major effort intended to improve consumer education by using a combination of advertising techniques to attract public attention. USDA also has introduced a labeling program that requires inclusion of instructions for safe food handling on retail packages of fresh meat.

Many programs, in addition to or in partnership with those of the federal government, provide guidance and education on food safety. University extension programs address all aspects of food safety education from the producer to the consumer. Topics include the development and implementation of HACCP programs, audits of processing plants, process control, and safe food handling by food service workers. Extension personnel also respond to food safety questions asked by food producers, processors, distributors, retailers, and consumers.

Private Efforts

Professional societies such as the American Dietetic Association, the Society for Nutrition Education, and the IFT offer a wide variety of food safety and consumer education materials. For example, they offer training and continuing education courses, videos, brochures, and textbooks.

The primary mission of not-for-profit organizations, such as the International Food Information Council (IFIC) and the Food Allergy Network (FAN), is to provide educational information about foods to consumers, media, industry, and policymakers. Conferences, media guidebooks, videos, publications in cooperation with government agencies, and resource-rich Web pages are some of the technical and educational tools that IFIC and FAN use. The Food and Drug Law Institute (FDLI) seeks to improve public health by providing a neutral forum to examine the laws, regulations, and policies related to foods. FDLI sponsors courses, conferences, publications, and videos to accomplish this goal.

Trade associations host meetings, symposia, and workshops that address the food safety issues of producers, processors, retailers, and the food service industry. Associations such as the NFPA, AMI, the NCBA, the NPPC, GMA, FMI, the NRA, and the National Meat Association provide an array of programs to assist their members with food safety matters. Many food companies provide toll-free telephone numbers and Web addresses for consumers to pose questions and concerns regarding the safety of their products. Many companies also distribute brochures or leaflets with information about food product safety and safe food handling practices, which is sometimes incorporated in materials such as recipes and advertisements.

CONSUMER RESPONSIBILITY AND PERCEPTIONS

Public perceptions about food risks shape personal and household behaviors and create demand for or acceptance of governmental actions related to food safety (See Box 2-1). Perceptions of foodborne hazards by the public often differ from those of the scientific community. For many years, risks posed by chemicals in food have concerned the consumer more than the expert, while the reverse is true for microbial hazards (Wolf, 1992). Those disparate views seem to arise from the values, needs, and priorities that the different sectors apply as they judge the acceptability of risks. It has been suggested that the criteria used by the public to judge the acceptability of risks include such risk attributes as familiarity, choice (whether the risk is voluntary or imposed), controllability, memorability, dread, immediacy, detectability, and equity of the distribution of risks and benefits. The levels of dread and the degree to which a risk is voluntary culminate in an "outrage" factor, which has been used to predict the acceptability of a risk (Groth, 1991; NRC, 1989; Sandman, 1987; Scherer, 1991; Slovic, 1986, 1987; Slovic et al., 1979).

Cultural factors also play a role in public responses to food safety issues. Public acceptance of a risk and demands for protection have been described as related to values and views associated with such things as freedom of choice, government regulation, understanding of technology, credibility of science, preference for homemade or natural foods, and attribution of risks to fate (Dale and Wildavsky, 1991; Douglas, 1985; Douglas and Wildavsky, 1982; Fitchen, 1987; NRC, 1989).

BOX 2-1.   Public Perceptions About Food Risks

Alan Levy, chief of the FDA's Consumer Studies Branch of the Office of Scientific Analysis and Support, sees a striking difference between consumer concerns and consumer behavior when it comes to safe food handling. From 1988 to 1993, research results showed consumer concern about food safety increased, while unsafe food handling practice by consumers also increased. Levy suggests several reasons for this "disconnect." For the last 30 years, he says, a dominant theme has been that we have the safest food supply in the world. Consumers have internalized this message and believe that a few remaining problems can be fixed by government controls, so that personal behavior has little effect. Failures that occur in processing plants and restaurants are likely to be far more newsworthy than sporadic cases of illness, and some consumers might not recognize problems caused by their own actions in their own homes. Focus group studies of the dangers of *Vibrio vulnificus* and the consumption of raw oysters reveals that many people were knowledgeable about the risks, considered themselves "experts," and felt that they knew how to control the risks. Even people who are fairly knowledgeable about food safety issues often have serious misconceptions about foodborne illness and its consequences. If the public does not see this as a serious problem, there will be little sense of urgency to change behavior. One way to break through "is to give people a better picture of the magnitude of food safety problems and challenge people's understanding of themselves as experts." Levy says new data from the FoodNet surveillance system "may be the best way to challenge people's understanding of themselves as experts."
SOURCE: Adapted from *Changing Strategies: Changing Behavior* June 12–13, 1997. (USDA, FDA, CDC)

Consumer food handling practices are a critical control point in the management of food safety issues, especially hazards from pathogenic microorganisms. Yet many consumers in the United States fail to follow recommended practices, as indicated by surveys in which 26 percent of respondents reported not washing cutting boards after cutting raw meat, 50 percent said that they ate raw or undercooked eggs, 23 percent reported eating raw clams or oysters, and 23 percent reported eating undercooked hamburgers (Appendix C).

Lack of knowledge of safe food handling practices can contribute to risky practices, and traditional rules about safe food handling practices are incomplete with respect to some food safety hazards, such as risks posed by eating a raw egg or a rare hamburger. A 1996 study found that 98 percent of respondents knew that meat and poultry could contain harmful bacteria and 75 percent knew that harmful bacteria could be present in dairy and egg products. However, fewer than half the respondents knew that harmful bacteria could be present on fruits and vegetables. In spite of this, a 1997 survey found that 88 percent of Americans believed they were taking precautionary steps in food handling practices to prevent foodborne illness (Partnership for Food Safety Education, 1997a).

Recent research indicates that general misconceptions might explain the failure of many consumers to practice safe food handling: they believe that foodborne illness is limited to fairly mild gastrointestinal distress that is experienced shortly after eating, that food safety problems can be seen or smelled, and foodborne illness is viewed as something that happens to others and not to them (Partnership for Food Safety Education, 1997a).

Aggressive efforts are essential to promote awareness of the risks from foodborne illness and to increase the public's use of safe food handling practices. Representatives who spoke to the committee agreed with the importance of this task:

> *"I want my child to come home from school and remind me to follow food safety practices in the home the same way my nieces and nephews instruct me on why and how I should recycle my trash" (Rhona Applebaum, NFPA, personal communication to committee, April 1998).*

Partnerships between government agencies and trade associations, professional organizations, and public interest groups are significant initial steps in instituting an aggressive campaign to promote consumers' understanding of actions to reduce foodborne risks. The Partnership for Food Safety Education developed the "Fight BAC" campaign, an ambitious and far-reaching education effort to educate the public about safe food handling (Partnership for Food Safety Education, 1997b). The campaign uses graphics and a public service announcement to promote four key principles for safe food handling: wash hands and surfaces often, prevent cross-contamination, cook foods to proper temperatures, and refrigerate foods promptly. The campaign builds on past efforts of government agencies and other groups to promote safe food handling practices by the public.

Adoption and use of those recommended practices will not be easily achieved. Individual behaviors are influenced by experience and by views of other important people in one's life, as well as by information received from experts. People are selective in their attention to risks, and their beliefs often change only slowly. Awareness of food risks and knowledge about recommended practices might not be reflected in behavior changes and risk reduction.

Safe food handling practices involve everyday behaviors that have many different dimensions and involve multiple resources, such as equipment, time, and skills. Changing those practices is more complicated than changing consumer preferences from one brand of a product to another, as is the aim in product advertising. Changing behaviors related to food handling is more complex than changing some other health behaviors, such as seatbelt use.

The time, attention, energy, and resources needed for the ambitious goal of reshaping the public's food handling practices must be recognized. Adequate resources and sustained program efforts over several years will be needed. Many causes compete for the public's attention, and professionals and community-based volunteers who are called on to assist in the campaign have competing demands on their time. A recent statement by Dr. C. Everett Koop in an independent panel report on food safety education emphasizes the vital importance of the goal: "Putting the country's resources behind public education on safe food handling is not only logical, it is absolutely essential. Now is the time to give this investment in basic information and public awareness the attention it deserves." (Partnership for Food Safety Education, 1997a).

THE ROLE OF MEDIA-GOVERNMENT PARTNERSHIPS IN FOOD SAFETY EDUCATION

The popular media—television, print, and radio—have long been the primary channels for communicating food-related science to the public and they play a major role in shaping public attitudes toward food safety. Media interest in this subject continues to grow. One three-month survey of coverage of diet, nutrition, and food safety issues by 38 local and national news outlets found that discussions of foodborne illness accounted for about 10 percent of all topical discussions, nearly twice the figure in 1995 (IFIC, 1998).

Although increased media coverage of foodborne illness might be beneficial in drawing attention to serious issues, it can also contribute to consumer fear and result in misunderstandings about real and perceived risks. Experts are sometimes misquoted, information can be misinterpreted or presented out of context, and hype-prone headlines can quickly give a benign article an alarming spin. To the public, perception *is* reality; thus regulatory agencies and government officials cannot afford to avoid media contact or to remain silent when food safety debates emerge, regardless of whether the perceived danger is real or imagined.

RESEARCH AND DEVELOPMENT

Federal Research Activities

Most federal research on food safety is conducted or administered by the following agencies:

- USDA: Agricultural Research Service (ARS), Cooperative State Research, Education and Extension Service (CSREES), and the Economic Research Service;
- DHHS: FDA and National Institutes of Health (NIH);
- Department of Commerce: NMFS;
- EPA; and,
- The Department of Defense.

Food safety is a comparatively small part of the total research and development efforts of these agencies. Food safety is not at the top of the research agenda in any of the agencies, whether measured by budget share, staff, or management emphasis. Although definitive data are difficult to obtain, it appears that food safety does not dominate the agenda or the culture of the agencies; therefore food safety research is often difficult to defend and support, and it suffers during periods of shrinking budgets or crises that affect other items on the agenda.

Other federal agencies—such as CDC, APHIS, AMS, GIPSA, and FSIS— cooperate in research projects that use their infrastructure for data or sample collection. They also affect research through the development of improved diagnostic procedures, recognition of new problems, and through their surveillance and epidemiological activities.

The fragmented character and complexity of federal food safety research foster a culture of competition rather than collaboration among the agencies and scientists involved. It would require extraordinary efforts to develop and coordinate a federal food safety research agenda given the current organizational structure. The agencies recently established several interagency bodies or activities to coordinate research, for example, the ARS-FSIS annual workshop; a risk assessment consortium of FDA, USDA, EPA, and the University of Maryland; the USDA-university workshop on "Enhancing Cooperation in Food Safety Research and Education;" the FSIS Food Safety Research Working Group; and the National Science and Technology Council under the Office of Science and Technology Policy made up of representatives of FSIS, CSREES, ARS, FDA, CDC, and EPA. These efforts at coordination appear to have grown out of the increasing national concern about food safety. Both increased research and increased coordination of research are important components of the *Food Safety from Farm to Table: National Food-Safety Initiative* (Appendix C).

Research priorities and implementation strategies for common goals tend to be determined from an agency perspective rather than as part of an integrated national program. For example, the need for increased surveillance of and epidemiological research on human illness and human pathogens in farm animals is generally recognized. In response, CDC, USDA, and FDA are cooperating with several states to establish a national infrastructure (FoodNet) for household-level studies of human illness. The USDA's APHIS has a national infrastructure for conducting epidemiological studies of animal health, which has been used for on-farm surveillance and field studies on pathogens. This APHIS responsibility has now been assigned to FSIS, and the funding has been reduced. The FSIS strategy is to contract with other federal and state agencies for on-farm epidemiological studies that can be conducted without a national infrastructure. USDA was attempting to consolidate its food safety efforts, but it has reduced its critical capacity and scientific base in this field.

FSIS does not have research authority. ARS, a research agency, has the intramural character and top-down management structure to respond quickly to some of the changing needs of FSIS by redirecting, expanding, or sustaining projects or programs. FSIS formally communicates its research needs and priorities to ARS once a year. In addition, scientists and management from the two agencies jointly review work in progress and plans for the future at an annual workshop.

USDA separates its intramural (ARS and ERS) and extramural (CSREES) research into different agencies even though most other departments combine intramural and extramural programs. The extramural programs support networks of scientists at universities throughout the nation. These networks leverage federally funded research with the intellectual and physical resources of the universities and with state and private research funds. Some university research is investigator-initiated in response to federal programs (such as those of NIH and the CSREES National Research Initiative) designed to bring science to food safety research. Some is in the form of grants or contracts structured to meet the immediate research needs of regulatory agencies. Much of the university research funded by state or private funds is targeted at specific state, regional, or commodity problems that have national importance.

Not all research related to food safety is identified as such. For example, although NIH does not have a research program directed specifically at food safety, it conducts research on foodborne diseases within the overall NIH mission of research to understand disease processes in humans and devise intervention strategies to improve human health. NIH has provided much of the basic knowledge about the microorganisms that cause foodborne diseases. That basic knowledge provides openings for NIH, other agencies, and industry to conduct research and to develop diagnostic tests or other control strategies. Thus, NIH research on microorganisms provides many of the strategic underpinnings for much of the targeted food safety research conducted by other organizations. In the aggregate, the NIH budget for research related to food safety is slightly below the USDA food safety research budget (Appendix E). In contrast with USDA, the NIH extramural program is larger than the intramural one. NIH research is not well-integrated with research at regulatory agencies that are assigned specific authority for food safety.

University research is largely supported by private industry, under grants or contracts with private companies or commodity to conduct intramural research on food safety. The outcomes of the research are, for the most part, proprietary and are not available to federal agencies or the public. Although information from the research is not usually distributed as widely as that generated by public funds, the industrial research is a large and essential component of the national food safety research effort.

Application of New Technology

The current system is slow to adopt new technologies that can improve food safety due to potential for harm if inadequately evaluated. For example, approval of irradiation was complicated by the 1958 congressional decision that irradiation be regulated as a food additive (rather than as a process) in spite of the lack of evidence that irradiation added anything to the product (Olson, 1998). Subsequent extensive research in both the United States and other countries documented that irradiation is a safe and effective means of reducing the risk of exposure to foodborne pathogens, and contributed to the development of procedures for the irradiation of foods. FDA approved the use of this technology for spices in 1982, for controlling porkborne trichinosis in 1985, and for poultry in 1990. It established the maximal doses of radiation that could be used in these applications and required that irradiated products be so labeled. FSIS established rules for implementing irradiation technology after FDA granted its approval for pork and poultry. These approvals also established the minimal dose of radiation that could be used, specified the design of the required label, and established requirements for record-keeping and inspection.

There has been little demand for irradiated pork and poultry in the ensuing years. In the absence of any economic incentives for the industry to adopt the technology, there has been comparatively little education of consumers or producers about the process, and some individuals and groups have objected to any educational activities that might be seen as promoting the use of irradiation (FMI, 1998b). In 1997, FDA approved irradiation of beef and more intensive use of irradiation for pork and poultry, and FSIS is establishing procedures to implement the technology in these applications.

Once the procedures are established by FSIS, adoption of the technology will depend on consumer acceptance and other economic incentives to the industry. Among the economic incentives for industry to adopt and promote irradiation are the destruction of *E. coli* O157:H7, an adulterant of ground beef and other foods that can result in product recalls, and extension of the shelf-life of products. These effects also benefit consumers. Consumer acceptance and demand are increasing somewhat; broad implementation will require substantial new investments in irradiation facilities and further development of FDA-approved packaging materials. However, it seems unlikely that irradiation of foods will increase markedly unless there is a change in the magnitude of educational effort on the principles, efficacy, and safety of irradiation.

INTERNATIONAL DIMENSIONS

Any assessment of the US food safety system must consider the effects of activities outside the United States. Food is vital everywhere; countries other than the United States also take measures to protect the safety of food consumed domestically. The dramatic increase in international food trade means that the diet in most countries includes food produced abroad. This can be enriching, both culturally and nutritionally, but it presents increasing challenges for regulators in the United States and elsewhere. Threats to food safety do not respect international boundaries, so all countries exporting to the United States must be included in a food safety system that assures that risks associated with imported foods do not undermine the safety of domestically produced foods. Although cultural and legal differences among countries are significant issues when considering the adoption of measures from other countries, the efforts of close trading partners to the United States can be instructive.

The scientific bases for food safety decision-making are generally published in the open literature and available internationally. The responses of foreign countries to threats faced in the United States might yield useful lessons for US regulators. The committee heard about and reviewed recent efforts by other governments to reform their food safety systems in response to recent concerns about disease transmission and food contamination (Appendix D).

Food Safety Efforts of Other Countries

Canada, Australia, and New Zealand have recently undertaken efforts to reform decentralized and fragmented food safety systems. The European Community and the United Kingdom have both taken preliminary steps toward centralizing their food safety efforts. Although the incentives for these efforts vary from country to country, there appear to be some common purposes, which include providing a single, consolidated focus for food safety efforts to enhance efficiency and reduce costs, responding to contemporary scientific developments, making use of external expertise, and fostering foreign markets for domestic food products. Steps have been taken largely to promote the interests of producers, processors, and regulators rather than the public health, but some health benefits will accrue.

Canada

In 1997, the Canadian government consolidated all federally mandated food inspection and quarantine services into a single federal food inspection agency, the Canadian Food Inspection Agency (CFIA). The goals of CFIA are to harmonize standards among federal, provincial, and municipal governments; to improve import and export controls and efficiency; and to enhance the international competitiveness of Canadian industry and products. As of April 1998, the agency was developing an integrated inspection system, streamlined food inspection, and a plant and animal health strategy for the entire food chain from input materials through production to retail sale and consumer use (CFIA, 1997, 1998). It has delegated the inspection activity to local governments.

Other Countries and Cooperatives

In July 1996, Australia and New Zealand established the Australian New Zealand Food Authority to develop and implement uniform food standards for the two countries. The European Commission has established the Food and Veterinary Office to monitor food hygiene, veterinary health, and plant health legislation within the European Union, and has embraced risk-assessment procedures to establish control priorities. In the United Kingdom, where food safety responsibility is divided between the Department of Health and the Ministry of Agriculture, Fisheries and Food, the government in January 1998 proposed the establishment of an independent Food Standards Agency (MAFF, 1998).

Increasing trade in food has also produced opportunities for international cooperation in the evaluation of and response to food safety challenges. The Codex Alimentarius is perhaps the best known inter-governmental effort (FAO/WHO, 1997). Although the Codex is driven by a powerful desire to achieve uniform regulatory standards in the interests of trade, it also contributes to an elevation of food safety standards in many countries. In doing so, the Codex and similar efforts assist US regulators in keeping imported food relatively safe.

US Regulation of Imported Foods

The continuing internationalization of the US food supply poses a singular challenge. As food imports into the United States have increased dramatically in the last generation, questions have been raised about the government's ability to ensure the safety of imported foods (GAO, 1998). The production, processing, and shipment of food produced in the United States can, in theory, be subject to government monitoring from field to dinner table, but imported food is not subject to such oversight.

Theoretically, Congress could forbid the importation not only of food that does not meet all domestic standards but also of food whose production is not subject to oversight by US officials in the same fashion as if it were produced domestically. Such a policy would require exporting countries to allow regular inspections by US inspectors; this would be politically unlikely and very expensive. Accordingly, the United States has adopted different strategies for protecting the safety of imported food.

Both FDA and USDA take the position, as their laws require, that imported food meet the same standards of labeling, composition, and safety as domestically produced food. That goal seems obvious, but it is not easily achieved. However, a recent General Accounting Office (GAO) report found that FDA and USDA have adopted rather different approaches (GAO, 1998).

FDA relies primarily on physical inspection and chemical analysis of imported food under its jurisdiction, using a sampling system that results in examination of 3 percent of all imported lots (GAO, 1998). It also relies on its knowledge of, or agreements reached with, the regulatory systems of the countries providing imports, focusing more port-of-entry attention on foods from countries where food safety controls are thought to fall short of US requirements. FDA is authorized to refuse admission to foods that appear to be adulterated, misbranded, or manufactured under unsanitary conditions; FDA may request that US Customs provide samples for inspection. FDA, with host-country agreement, occasionally undertakes some overseas inspections of production and processing facilities.

GAO questions whether FDA is ensuring that imported foods meet domestic safety standards. Domestic food inspections by FDA have become less frequent in the last decade, just as its examinations of imported shipments have not kept pace with the growth of imports. More important, many pathogens and chemical contaminants that pose health risks are not readily detectable with the means available to FDA at the port-of-entry.

USDA follows a rather different approach. An exporting country can seek official certification of its domestic control system for meat and poultry as "equivalent" to that of the United States. Certification of equivalence is based on an on-site review of its performance. In cooperation with US Customs, USDA refuses imports of meat and poultry from any country whose domestic regulatory system is not judged "equivalent" to its own. Once a country's system is determined to be equivalent (which requires that it include the same sort of carcass-by-carcass examination that historically has characterized USDA's inspection approach), imports are accepted without inspection of individual shipments. About 40 countries are approved to export meat products and five to export poultry products to the United States (9 CFR 327.2(b); 381.196(b)).

The different systems of scrutiny of imports used by FDA and USDA largely mirror their different approaches to domestically produced food as is required since they must document domestic equivalence. History and statutory mandate, rather than scientific rationale, lead USDA to demand carcass-by-carcass inspection domestically. FDA, with its smaller budget, aspires to examine imports thoroughly but cannot do so. Neither approach is based on a rigorous assessment of risk. The major outbreak of foodborne illness traced to raspberries from Guatemala could not have been prevented by port-of-entry inspection, even if an inspection had taken place.

International competition and the desire for export markets are primary factors leading to changes in food safety systems. As free trade agreements have been signed, trade disputes have increasingly focused on technical standards and inspection requirements. Other countries have been forced to revise domestic standards to establish equivalence with trading partners. The United States may also need to be concerned about the relationship of our food safety system to international trade. One important concern is that our system be scientifically grounded so that its requirements are recognized as legitimate protections of safety rather than as trade barriers. This report does not address issues of the safety of foods and food products exported, but exports are a major component of many food companies. Thus, new approaches must improve food safety at home and meet requirements abroad.

SUMMARY FINDINGS: The Current US System for Food Safety

- Has many of the attributes of an effective system;
- is a complex, interrelated activity involving government at all levels, the food industry from farm and sea to table, universities, the media, and the consumer;
- is moving toward a more science-based approach with HACCP and with risk-based assessment;
- is limited by statute in implementing practices and enforcement that are based in science; and
- is fragmented by having 12 primary federal agencies involved in key functions of safety: monitoring, surveillance, inspection, enforcement, outbreak management, research, and education.

3

The Changing Nature of Food Hazards: Cause for Increasing Concern

There have been dramatic changes in the US food supply. These changes have contributed to recent outbreaks of infectious foodborne illness, which in turn led to the request for this committee to examine aspects of the US food safety system. The committee recognizes the growing concern for controlling the microbiological hazards related to food, but believes that government attention must also be addressed to chemical and physical hazards. This chapter is organized in two parts: the first describes major changes that affect the epidemiology of infectious foodborne disease, and the second describes examples of potential chemical hazards which have emerged in part from some of the same changes in the food supply. Physical hazards related to food are addressed briefly at the end of this chapter.

CHANGES THAT AFFECT THE EPIDEMIOLOGY OF FOODBORNE DISEASE

Recent outbreaks of foodborne disease caused by many different pathogens and involving a variety of food products have been the subject of headlines, but it is unclear whether the incidence of foodborne disease has increased over the last generation. The major reason for the uncertainty is that the lack of a national foodborne-disease surveillance system has prevented the study of trends in disease rates. What is clear is that factors affecting the potential safety of the nation's food supply have changed dramatically over the last generation and

51

justify concern that the incidence of foodborne disease is high and may be increasing.

At least five trends contribute to the possible increase in foodborne disease: changes in diet, the increasing use of commercial food services, new methods of producing and distributing food, new or re-emerging infectious foodborne agents, and the growing number of people at high risk for severe or fatal foodborne diseases.

Diet

Annual food expenditures in the United States, as a share of disposable personal income, decreased from 14 percent to 11 percent from 1970 to 1996 (Putnam and Allshouse, 1997). No industrialized nation spends a smaller share of its wealth on food than the United States. For much of the population, readily available food is more varied and more affordable than ever before. For example, in the 1960s, an average US grocery store had fewer than 7,000 food items available. Today, an average US grocery store sells about 30,000 food items (FMI, 1997b), and over 12,000 new products are introduced each year (New Product News, 1998).

During this time when relative costs of the US food supply are decreasing, per capita consumption of many foods has changed substantially. Public health efforts to promote a "heart-healthy" diet have helped to boost the consumption of fresh fruits and vegetables. On a per capita basis, in 1995, Americans ate about 31 lb more commercially grown vegetables, including potatoes and sweet potatoes, and 24 lb more fresh fruit than in 1970 (Putnam and Allshouse, 1997). As the consumption and variety of produce have increased, so has the importation of produce from developing countries. The General Accounting Office estimates that in 1995 one-third of all fresh fruit consumed in the United States was imported (GAO, 1998). Food imports have increased both because of lower production costs in foreign countries and because of consumer demand for year-round supplies of fruits and vegetables that have limited growing seasons in the United States. For example, 17 percent of cantaloupes, 52 percent of green onions, 36 percent of cucumbers, and 34 percent of tomatoes sold in the United States in 1996 were grown in Mexico (Osterholm et al., 1998). Seasonally, as much as 79 percent of a particular commodity consumed in this country has been raised in Mexico alone, and the percentage of produce from other developing countries consumed here is growing rapidly. Fresh produce items were the leading vehicle associated with foodborne disease outbreaks in Minnesota from 1990 to 1996, accounting for almost one-third of all outbreaks (Osterholm et al., 1998). This percentage is higher than that available from national foodborne disease surveillance data and possibly reflects more active surveillance in that state.

Other trends in the United States are the decreasing consumption of beef and the increased consumption of chicken and seafood. In 1970, the average

American consumed 79 lb of beef, 27 lb of chicken, and 12 lb of fish and shellfish; in 1996, annual per capita consumptions were 64, 50 and 15 lb, respectively (Putnam and Allshouse, 1997). Contamination of red meat with *Salmonella* and *Escherichia coli* O157:H7 remains important, but the risk posed by chicken as a vehicle for *Campylobacter* and *Salmonella* has grown substantially (Consumers Union, 1998).

Cultural changes affect not only what Americans eat, but also where they eat and how their food is prepared. Increasingly, Americans have time-pressured lifestyles. Saving time and effort in shopping for and preparing food will continue to be important for many Americans. Households with a single parent or two working adults often face particular pressures in food shopping and meal preparation that can affect food selection and safety (Federal Coordinating Council for Science, Engineering, and Technology, 1993). Cookbook sales and television cooking shows demonstrate that cooking is popular, but there seems to be decreased interest in ordinary daily home food preparation and, with most adults working, a lack of role models in the kitchen. Reductions in time for and interest in home food preparation also result in changed food patterns, fewer homemade dishes, more reliance on leftovers, increased purchase of prepared or convenience foods, and frequent eating away from home (FMI, 1997a).

With less time spent in the kitchen and greater availability of high-quality, ready-to-eat dishes and convenience items, Americans' food preparation skills are diminishing. As a result, appreciation of simple but critical food safety techniques, such as washing hands and utensils and storing foods at optimal temperatures, has likely diminished.

Individual food tastes and preparation styles are brought to the United States from around the world, and the increasing ethnic diversity of the American population may affect food safety in several ways. Different ethnic groups have different concerns and practices regarding food safety, and this could affect the activities of immigrants as food preparers at home and in the workplace. New food risks can arise as immigrant populations adapt traditional preferences and practices to their new environment. Food safety education programs should consider the food beliefs and practices of various cultural groups.

Although data show a rise in perceived risk of foodborne illness among consumers (Alan Levy, FDA, Food Safety Survey Data, communication to committee, June 1998), attitudes do not always translate into improved food-handling practices. Over half of all shoppers report washing their hands and/or food preparation surfaces, yet only 28 percent know that cooking temperatures are critical and that foods should be refrigerated promptly (FMI, 1998a). A recent Food and Drug Administration (FDA) study found that many US consumers still eat undercooked hamburger meat and raw eggs (Alan Levy, FDA, 1998 Food Safety Survey Data, communication to committee, June 1998).

Commercial Food Services

The percentage of the food dollar spent on food consumed away from home has risen dramatically over the last three decades. In 1970, only 34 percent of our food dollars were spent eating away from home. In contrast, in 1996, 46 percent of our food dollars were spent for meals and snacks prepared outside the home (Putnam and Allshouse, 1997). Institutional feeding sites serve a wide range of people—from very young children in child care centers to the elderly—in congregate sites for meals, alternative-care centers, and nursing homes. Meals are also prepared as takeout foods from supermarkets and convenience stores; many of these meals include one or more cold food items, such as delicatessen sandwiches and salads that require extensive food handling and are not cooked before consumption. These changes have led to an increase in the number of people handling food and the potential for an increase in the transmission of foodborne diseases from food handlers to consumers.

The average food handler in this country earns the minimum wage, lacks sick leave and other health benefits, and has very limited opportunities for advancement. These jobs are filled by people with few employment opportunities and low economic status, conditions that may be related to a high incidence of intestinal diseases and low rates of routine hand washing. Recent evidence from Minnesota demonstrates the increased risk of food handler associated transmission of *Salmonella typhimurium*; this finding was documented because *Salmonella* isolates in Minnesota undergo molecular characterization and epidemiologic investigation (Osterholm et al., 1998). Food handlers in other areas of the United States probably play a similar role in the transmission of *Salmonella* and other enteric agents.

Methods of Production and Distribution

The changing availability and sources of our food supply have brought changes in methods of producing and distributing food. Today, large manufacturing plants can process quantities and types of products that two decades ago would have required many smaller plants. Although the ability to control possible hazards increases when there are fewer plants, the potential for larger outbreaks—even if product contamination is minimal—is evident. Thousands of people become ill during such outbreaks. For example, contamination of tanker trucks with nonpasteurized liquid eggs and subsequent use of those trucks to haul pasteurized ice cream mix most likely led to the largest documented outbreak of salmonellosis in the United States (Hennessy et al., 1996). That outbreak showed that even sporadic low level contamination of a single product can result in a major epidemic of foodborne illness because of the quantity of product consumed.

In the spring of 1998, a cereal produced by the largest generic label manufacturer of cereal in the United States caused a national outbreak of *Salmonella agona* infection. Outbreaks such as this can be difficult to detect because contamination of the product is sporadic and the product is marketed widely.

The driving forces of globalization, advanced technology, and economic competitiveness have dramatically affected the structure and practices of livestock and poultry production. Herds, flocks, and other populations of food animals, including fish and seafood, are increasingly concentrated in fewer and larger production units. The traditional farmstead model of the past, often characterized by multiple species and small numbers of food animals reared on a single farm, has been replaced by specialized, large-scale production systems. For example, from 1994 to 1995, the number of US hog operations decreased from 207,980 to 182,700, but both the inventory of hogs and the total number of hogs produced increased during the same time (NASS, 1995). That mirrors the general agribusiness trend, and the restructuring continues.

New or Re-emerging Infectious Foodborne Agents

The role of new or re-emerging causes of foodborne diseases is well-recognized, but the size of the increase in risk is unknown. Emerging and re-emerging infections have been defined as new, recurring, or drug-resistant infections whose incidence in humans has increased in the last two decades or whose incidence threatens to increase in the near future (NRC, 1993). Recent examples of newly recognized agents are *E. coli* O157:H7, other pathogenic *E. coli*, *Cyclospora*, and *Cryptosporidium*. Old agents re-emerging in new vehicles or product streams include *Salmonella enteritidis* in eggs and hepatitis A virus in produce. Finally, there have been recent increases in antimicrobial resistance of pathogens, such as *S. typhimurium* DT104 and *Campylobacter jejuni* in humans, which have been attributed to the use of antimicrobial agents in food animals (Osterholm et al., 1998).

The frequently cited annual estimates of foodborne disease (up to 81 million cases) and 9,000 associated deaths are based on assumptions that do not necessarily reflect the current national foodborne disease problem. Those estimates must be qualified for two reasons. First, no comprehensive population-based studies of gastrointestinal illness in the community have attempted to determine what proportion of these illnesses is due to consumption of contaminated food and what proportion is from other sources. Second, foodborne illness can cause clinical conditions not characterized by gastrointestinal symptoms, such as congenital toxoplasmosis, hemolytic uremic syndrome, salmonella-associated septicemia, and invasive *Listeria* infections (Morris and Potter, 1997). In the absence of comprehensive estimates of foodborne disease incidence, the only data available are those from the FoodNet program.

Data from FoodNet—an effort sponsored by the Centers for Disease Control and Prevention, the US Department of Agriculture, FDA, and the health departments of California, Connecticut, Georgia, Minnesota, and Oregon—have demonstrated that the incidence of diarrheal illness in the United States is about 1.4 episodes per person per year, or some 370 million episodes of diarrhea each year. Population-based studies of diarrheal disease conducted from 1948 through 1971 in Ohio and Michigan demonstrate an incidence of about one episode per person per year (Osterholm et al., 1998). The reason for the apparent 40 percent difference between these estimates is unclear, but it is evident that the problem is large. If only 25 percent of diarrheal disease is food-related, the burden of foodborne diarrheal disease in the United States far exceeds current estimates.

Studies conducted by FoodNet suggest that fewer than 2 percent of the cases of diarrheal illness in the United States can be attributed to *Salmonella*, *Campylobacter*, *Shigella*, *E. coli* O157:H7, and *Yersinia* (Osterholm et al., 1998). Little information is available on the role of other pathogens, including newly recognized agents such as Shiga toxin-producing *E. coli* other than O157:H7, *Cryptosporidium*, and *Cyclospora,* and previously established pathogens such as Norwalk-like viruses, *Clostridium perfringens*, *Staphylococcus aureus*, *Bacillus cereus,* and hepatitis A virus. Until additional studies elucidate the role of the recognized pathogens in foodborne disease, we can only speculate about the occurrence of new or unrecognized pathogens.

Populations at High Risk for Severe or Fatal Foodborne Disease

The risk of foodborne disease is related to several factors, including the presence and dose of a pathogen or toxin in food, the virulence of the pathogen or toxin, the mechanisms of transmission, and the susceptibility of a host. Many factors influence susceptibility to infection and the severity of disease, including age, the use of immunosuppressive agents, and disease states that increase immunosuppression.

Young children are more likely than adults to develop illness from selected pathogens, and children have been high-profile victims of several foodborne disease outbreaks in recent years. Young children today are likely to be exposed to a broader range of foodborne diseases than was true a generation ago, because families eat out or take prepared food home more often and children receive more community and out-of-home care at younger ages.

Elderly persons are particularly susceptible to illness from foodborne disease, and the number of the elderly in the United States is increasing rapidly. From 1965 to 1995, the number of Americans aged 65 years or older grew by 82 percent. As the 75 million persons in the "baby boomer" generation (equaling one-third of the population) age, the United States can expect one-fifth of the population to be over the age of 65 within the next three decades (US Census Bureau, 1997).

As the population ages, the incidence of cancer and other chronic diseases is likely to increase. These diseases will require an increased use of chemotherapeutic regimens, drugs to deal with rejection of solid organ transplantations, and antimicrobial drugs that have important effects on the normal (and beneficial) bacterial flora of the intestinal tract. Together, these factors predispose people to both the occurrence and the serious outcomes of foodborne disease. The increasing number of people with immunosuppressive diseases, such as human immunodeficiency virus, also contributes to the public health importance of food safety.

CHANGES IN CHEMICAL HAZARDS ASSOCIATED WITH THE FOOD SUPPLY

Changes in our society and our food supply have raised new concerns about food chemical safety. Some of the changes that have raised new concerns about foodborne infectious disease are also affecting how government agencies carry out the more familiar task of protecting the food supply from toxic chemical agents.

Foods are themselves a complex collection of naturally occurring chemicals that have nutritive, organoleptic, and pharmacological functions and occasionally toxic effects. Naturally occurring toxicants probably present risks second only to those imposed by microorganisms. These natural toxicants include seafood toxins and foodborne mycotoxins.

Other chemicals are introduced into foods intentionally or unintentionally. Intentionally added substances include food and color additives, flavors, enzymes, vitamins and minerals, and other ingredients that help to add value or characteristic properties or functions to a food. Because of broad public concern about synthetic chemicals, the toxicologic profiles of many of these synthetic components of food are much more complete than those of natural components of food. As a result, the risks posed by regulated food additives are generally better characterized than those of many naturally occurring substances.

Unintentional additives can include environmental or industrial contaminants as well as some substances used in food production but not intended to be part of the food. The migration of food production substances into the final product is generally very low, but must be carefully regulated to ensure safety. Examples include sanitizers used to keep food production surfaces safe, packaging materials used to keep food safe and fresh, pesticides used on crops and drugs used in animals to mitigate damage, disease, microbial toxin production, and general food losses. Environmental or industrial contaminants are not sanctioned but have the potential to enter the food chain. Examples of chemical contamination incidents are methyl mercury in fish, mistaken mixing of polybrominated biphenyls (a fire retardant) into animal feed, and leakage of ammonia refrigerant into frozen foods.

Some people are sensitive or allergic to chemical constituents that are harmless to the rest of the population. These allergic reactions are estimated to occur in 1 to 2 percent of adults and 5 to 8 percent of children. Although serious reactions are rare, it is estimated that several dozen deaths occur each year because of allergic reactions to food (Bock, 1992). More than 160 foods and food-related substances have been identified as being able to cause allergic reactions (ILSI, 1996). However, in the United States, more than 90 percent of allergic reactions appear to be caused by just eight food types: peanuts, tree nuts (such as walnuts, pecans, almonds, hazel nuts), crustacea (shrimp, lobster, and other shellfish), eggs, milk, soy, fish, and wheat (Hefle et al., 1996).

Consequently, the subject of chemical hazards in food is complex and includes consideration of potential risks that vary widely in scope and severity. Many chemical hazards associated with foods have been recognized only in the last century as advancements have been made in chemistry, toxicology, and risk assessment. Public concern over these hazards has grown in recent decades, in line with the increasing distrust of chemicals generally and of their use in the environment. Indeed, there have been episodes of chemical intoxication (usually arising out of accident or occupational exposure) with tragic consequences. Although most experts agree that the more serious hazards in the American food supply are not chemical but microbiological, public concern has demanded that proportionally more regulatory resources be applied to chemical hazards (IFT, 1989).

New Food Components

The American public's growing interest in the relationship between diet and health has led to an increased demand for foods or food constituents that not only have nutritive value but also hold promise for prevention or even treatment of disease. These products have been referred to as dietary supplements, functional foods, pharma-foods or nutraceuticals. In a recent study, more than two-thirds of surveyed households reported use of a vitamin, mineral, or herbal supplement within the previous six-month period (Hartman and New Hope, 1998). The Dietary Supplement Health and Education Act of 1994 eased restrictions on certain statements of nutrition support made for supplements and exempted them from the safety approval requirement applicable to conventional food additives. That legal change helped spur the growing market for supplements of all types, including herbal products, and raises food safety concerns. Some supplements and herbal products on the market may pose a risk of adverse health effects because they are not required to meet specified safety standards before being sold. They may thus contain varying amounts or unknown or inadequately characterized ingredients that can have pharmacological activity that has not been adequately characterized (for example, ephedrine in Chinese ma huang).

Food processors are examining relatively new sources of ingredients for more conventional functional properties. For example, gums and fibers such as konjac flour, tara gum, inulin, or psyllium fiber may provide bulk and texture to foods, yet have had limited food use in the United States. Potential broad use of these ingredients in domestic foods raises important safety questions: are there significant intestinal effects such as blockage or reduced transit times? Are there impacts on vitamin uptake from the intestinal tract or on osmotic balance? What are the potential allergy risks from increased exposure to plant-sourced materials? These are a few of the safety questions that may be raised when a new ingredient source is considered.

Food processors are also utilizing macronutrient substitutes, such as nonnutritive sweeteners and fat replacers in many food products. These macronutrient substitutes have potential value by lowering calories, sugar, or fat in food products. Because dietary quantities of these substitutes could be substantially higher than the amounts of typical food additives, the assessment of their safety can be particularly important as well as particularly difficult.

New Food Technologies

Modification of plants or animals via genetic engineering can improve yields and increase resistance to pests. This new technology might offer improvements in food safety through increased resistance to molds that produce food mycotoxins or through lower levels of allergenic proteins, fatty acids, or other undesirable components of food. However, there are important differences between countries in how food products from genetically modified organisms are regulated. Several products derived from genetic engineering have been declared safe by US regulators, but many European countries have either forbidden their sale or insisted on what marketers believe is disparaging labeling. Concerns about the safety of products from genetically engineered plants and animals are only partially resolved.

Food irradiation is not a new technology. Irradiation of fruits and vegetables decreases the risk of pathogens and extends shelf life. But as discussed in Chapter two, public concerns about the safety of irradiated food, fueled in part by a lack of consumer education, limits its use in the United States (FMI, 1998b). These concerns prompted the requirement that certain irradiated foods be labeled as such. The extent to which this labeling requirement has limited subsequent adoption of the process is unknown.

New or Re-emerging Toxic Agents

As the science of toxicology has progressed over the last 50 years, questions about the safety of chemicals in foods have become more sophisticated. When tougher safety standards are applied to new food chemicals or reapplied to old ones, new issues of toxicity emerge. The cycle of reevaluating safety standards began in the years after World War II when advances in the understanding of the mechanisms of carcinogenesis coincided with the increased use of rodent bioassays. The newly focused attention to carcinogens that ensued led Congress to pass the 1958 "Delaney clause" proscription of carcinogens. The focus on carcinogens in food continues to consume substantial testing and regulatory resources. Further advances in biomedical research have raised new concerns and new standards of safety that now address teratogenicity, reproductive toxicity, mutagenicity, hormonal effects, and immunotoxicity.

The effects of food constituents on hormonal function is of concern as medical research has indicated the importance of certain hormones in regulating diseases such as breast cancer and osteoporosis. This phenomenon, sometimes referred to as endocrine disruption, led Congress in 1996 to mandate special regulatory attention to the issue and inspired the Environmental Protection Agency (EPA) to convene an expert panel, the Endocrine Disrupter Screening and Testing Advisory Committee. That committee has attempted to define endocrine disrupters, determine analytical methods, and recommend how the disrupters should be regulated. Potential candidates for evaluation include constituents of some food packaging materials, pesticides, and natural food constituents, such as genestein in soy.

Some groups have recently asked whether chemical safety assessments provide adequate safety margins to protect children (Guzelian et al., 1992; NRC, 1993). That concern drawns attention because new pesticide legislation directs EPA to consider the aggregate risks posed by any pest control agent; that is, exposures should be assessed for all potential sources of a chemical and for other chemicals with a similar mechanism of action (21 USCA sec. 342(b)(2)(A)(ii)). Another concern is the emergence of evidence of subtle developmental and behavioral effects of relatively low concentrations of chemicals (for example, lead).

In summary, chemical hazards, as well as foodborne pathogens, present new and changing challenges to the food safety system. Federal food safety efforts will need full integration and sufficient support to meet these challenges.

Physical Hazards

The foods we consume begin as raw agricultural commodities grown in open fields or waters or raised in a variety of production facilities, such as barns, coops, pens, and feedlots. Rocks, stones, metal, wood, glass, and other physical objects can become part of raw ingredients. Further contamination can occur in the transport, processing, or distribution of foods because of equipment failure, accident, or negligence.

Foreign physical materials in foods can cause serious harm to consumers. Protective devices that remove or prevent physical hazards include metal detectors, magnets, sieves, traps, scalpers, and screens. Other effective means of protection are production plant policies against the use of glass, wood, or nonferrous metal where possible; employee training; quality audits of ingredient suppliers; and sensory tests.

Federal agencies have established "defect action levels" for natural or unavoidable defects that do not affect human health, such as stems or pits in fruits and vegetables, bone in mechanically deboned meats, and microscopic insect fragments, which are primarily of aesthetic concern and do not present a safety hazard.

SUMMARY FINDINGS: The Changing Nature of Food Hazards

- Changes in the risk of infectious foodborne disease are due primarily to:
    - changes in diet,
    - increasing use of commercial food service and in food eaten or prepared away from home,
    - new methods of producing and distributing food,
    - new or re-emerging infectious foodborne agents, and
    - the growing number of people at high risk for foodborne illnesses due to:
        — increasing number of elderly, and
        — increasing number of people with depressed immunity or resistance to infection.
- Changes in chemical hazards associated with the food supply must be monitored and evaluated; these include:
    - increased use of dietary supplements and herbal products without requirements to meet specified safety standards;
    - new food components that mimic attributes of traditional food components;
    - introduction of new food technologies and processes;
    - changes in presence of food toxins and additives, including unintentional food additives; and
    - presence of physical hazards associated with new technologies or sources of foods.

4

What Constitutes an Effective Food Safety System?

Earlier chapters have addressed the definition, historical significance, and current status of food safety in the United States as well as recent trends in and reasons for concern about foodborne hazards. This chapter turns to the features of an ideal food safety system and to a somewhat detailed description of its attributes. Constructing a model system establishes a benchmark that provides both a point of reference for judging actual systems and a goal to be achieved.

THE MISSION OF THE SYSTEM

There is universal agreement on the need for safe food, but no consensus on the means by which safe food is secured. The effectiveness of a food safety system begins with a clear, unified mission that focuses and integrates the varied needs and responsibilities of all stakeholders, gives the stakeholders a basis for achieving the goals of the system, and is broadly accepted.

The committee defines safe food as food that is wholesome, that does not exceed an acceptable level of risk associated with pathogenic organisms or chemical and physical hazards, and whose supply is the result of the combined activities of Congress, regulatory agencies, multiple industries, universities, private organizations, and consumers. The mission of a food safety system should be stated as an operational charge that uses and reflects that definition. The committee defines the mission as follows:

63

The mission of an effective food safety system is to protect and improve the public health by ensuring that foods meet science-based safety standards through the integrated activities of the public and private sectors.

The remainder of this chapter focuses on these matters. Activities that are implied in the definition and are incorporated in achieving the mission to ensure safe food include: adequate monitoring and surveillance; science-based research and development; incorporation of the tenets of risk analysis, including risk assessment, risk management, and risk communication; good practices in food production, processing, manufacturing, retail sale, transportation, preparation, and handling; and appropriate technical assistance and education. Box 4-1 provides a definition of science-based and related examples.

BOX 4-1.   What is the Meaning of Science-Based?

A science base for ensuring safe food encompasses many elements. When utilized, these elements improve the ability to identify, reduce, and manage risks; minimize occurrence of foodborne hazards; gather and utilize information; enhance knowledge; and improve overall food safety. Several examples of science-based actions that have been implemented in the US food safety system that are readily recognized as positive elements of the system include:

- Implementation of low-acid canned food processing technology, which reduces the risk of botulism;
- implementation of HACCP systems and risk assessment in decision-making;
- approval of irradiation technology for use in spices, pork, beef, poultry, fruits and vegetables;
- prohibition of the use of lead-based paints on utensils that come in contact with food;
- estimation of maximum allowable exposure levels to pesticides;
- development of standards for allowable practices associated with transport of foods following transport of pesticides in the same containers;
- use of labeling as a device to warn consumers who are sensitive to potential food allergens of the content of the allergen; and
- requirements that meat and poultry products at the retail level carry consumer information related to safe food handling practices.

While the approaches above are important successful science-based tools in food production and processing, these are only examples of implementation of the scientific basis for food safety. An effective food safety system also integrates science and risk analysis at all levels of the system, including food safety research, information and technology transfer, and consumer education.

Ensuring a system to provide safe food within the United States is a common goal, and legislative mandates should direct the components of that system. The mission should be focused on using public health resources and management to perform risk analysis and research and at the same time on optimizing coordination and planning of prevention, intervention, control, response, and communication mechanisms.

GENERAL ATTRIBUTES OF THE SYSTEM

An effective food safety system is an interdependent system composed of government agencies at all levels, businesses and other private organizations, consumers, and supporting players. The system is dynamic and aligned to the unified mission of improving food safety so as to maintain and improve the public's health and well-being.

Figure 4-1 depicts the interrelationships of an effective food safety system. Although the players have key, independent functions, they must implement many of their actions through strong partnerships. The system is built on the flexibility and adaptability of the players and on the nature and course of their

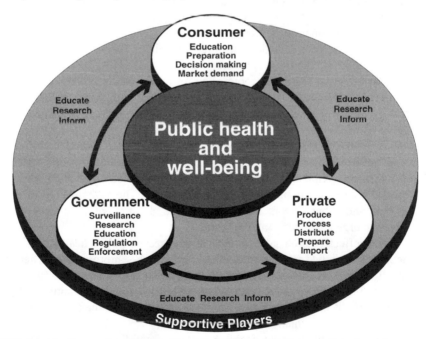

FIGURE 4-1. Attributes of an Effective Food Safety System: A Dynamic Interdependence. Partners in the system include government, private industry, and consumers. Supportive players, who are critical to the integration of the attributes of research, education, and information, include universities and colleges, the news media, and focused special interest organizations, among others.

relationships, and these affect their ability to prevent, identify, and resolve food safety issues in the most efficient, effective, and cost-beneficial manner. The system is responsive to the expedient issues of today but also evolves strategically to meet future challenges. It must be effective in both the domestic environment and the new global food environment, with increasing international trade.

The system is science-based with strong emphasis on risk analysis and the use of data. It is attentive to learning through the use of feedback loops and continuous improvement. Although responsiveness to and coordination of food safety crises are critical attributes, the system is designed to stress prevention and detection of emerging problems.

The system has adequate funding, is supported by strong research and education components, uses technology adequate to the task, and is integrated to achieve its mission. Statutory and regulatory authority promote the system's horizontal and vertical integration. Because integration is such a critical attribute, the system requires strong, centralized leadership. The system champions a culture of capacity building. With the transition toward a new scientific and risk-based foundation, agencies will encourage and fund retraining and further development of their employees, and they will initiate plans for the recruitment and retention of high-quality staff with the skills and knowledge to enhance the new system and its changing operations and focus. Capacity must also include consumer knowledge and practices, taking into account cultural sensitivities and practices.

An effective system is commensurate with today's driving forces, trends, and societal expectations. Partnerships will expand with the growing recognition that government cannot abandon our food safety problems to private industry and consumers.

The effective system stresses the inclusion of its players in their roles but also acknowledges the need for effective regulation, compliance, and enforcement. Although some of the roles will need to change, the system functions in an environment of trust and respect. The globalization of the food system and other factors that can increase the risk of foodborne incidents mandate urgency in adopting the system.

The effective food safety system is focused on public health, and its many actions are aligned to achieve a safer food supply, improve public health, and instill consumers' confidence in both the system and their role in improving it. Finally, the dynamic interconnectiveness also promotes the attainment by all of the players of both responsibility and accountability for making the food safety system perform optimally.

The following sections describe in more detail the attributes of an effective food safety system.

THE IMPORTANCE OF PARTNERING

Food safety is the responsibility of numerous and diverse stakeholders, and partnerships provide the links that are necessary to build a coordinated and cohesive framework for action. Partnerships can improve efficiency and provide a mechanism for information and technology transfer. Interaction and communication through partnerships lead to cooperation and collaboration among public and private interests. Partnerships can also help to integrate regulated activities with important non-regulatory components of the system.

Incentives can greatly influence and facilitate the building of effective partnerships. "Positive" incentives are often financial. "Negative" incentives can include the desire to avoid legal or regulatory action or media attention. Another incentive for partnerships can be the generation of new and useful information that improves production and processing capabilities simultaneously with improved control of risk.

The market is an important incentive for private industry. As global markets and domestic consumers expect safer food, safety itself can become a factor in differentiating products. Retailers can help to leverage this concept as brand names become associated with reduced risks.

Some factors, such as intellectual property issues, pose challenges to the establishment and maintenance of partnerships. These issues might become increasingly difficult in the future, as such sciences as the microbiology of food continue to advance rapidly.

Despite the challenges posed by the diversity of the players and changing priorities within the system, the potential realm of strong partnerships is large and includes all partners: government, the private sector, consumers, and support players, as shown in Figure 4-1. Partnerships should be formed and function in an open process that is independent and protected from political, economic, and social pressures. Partners must have clear delineations of responsibility and the authority to make decisions to meet responsibilities. They must have the resources to work together effectively. Successful partnerships are based on close, detailed, and accurate communication and collaboration.

THE ROLES OF GOVERNMENT PARTNERS

In the public sector, the federal government is in the best position to influence how the other components of the food safety system work together. Its actions, which often take the form of regulation, originate in federal food law. The federal government must guide the system with national food law that is clear, rational, and based on scientifically determined risk. A few principles form the basis for ideal food law, which can be conceptualized by the philosophical structure of food safety. This structure includes a process that is fair and open to participation by all without political, economic, or social pressures and that provides for adequate authority and budgetary considerations.

Legislation must be flexible and enforceable, and it must comprehensively address all aspects of the entire system from production to consumption. The authority and responsibility of the federal government and its interface with private and other partners must be well-articulated. Definition of a broad federal role is promoted by the similarities of food safety issues across states and demographic groups. Other levels of government have a role in shaping federal activities if they are to be effective in implementing national standards and in dealing separately with local issues.

With a sound food law in place, partnerships between the federal government and others in the system can establish a framework to provide several important functions. For instance, partnerships of federal, state, and local governments with industry, universities, private organizations, and consumers can ensure that the system is science-based and risk-focused, that surveillance and monitoring efforts provide sufficient information to maintain and improve effectiveness, that research and education efforts are properly focused, that regulation and enforcement are effective and consistent, that the system is responsive to new technologies and changing consumer needs, that a continuous process of evaluation can respond to the queries and problems of all stakeholders, and that resources are adequate and appropriately allocated throughout the system.

A Science-Based Foundation Using Risk Analysis

The scientific foundation for decision-making within a food safety system is risk analysis. The role of risk analysis in an effective food safety system is threefold: it provides a basis for identifying where resources should be allocated in the short term; it constitutes a mechanism for determining where public and private efforts should be directed in the long term, especially with respect to research and preventive measures; and it yields important information for estimating and analyzing the costs and benefits of policy alternatives.

The components of risk analysis—risk assessment, risk management, and risk communication—use interdependent approaches, methods, and models; none can function well in the absence of the others. Good risk communication is required for effective risk assessment and risk management. All components of risk analysis—scientific, economic, legal, behavioral, or other—require an environment that is independent of the derivation of policy and must be subject to agency leadership.

Focused risk assessment identifies risks that have the most important consequences for human health and (not always the same) shows where the most progress can be made with available resources. Scientific risk assessment should identify the risks associated with one or more possible actions, or risks associated with taking no action. Risk assessment is fairly well-developed for chemical hazards, such as pesticides, but not for foodborne pathogens.

Development of risk assessment for the complexity of such pathogens must be given high priority.

A pivotal component of risk analysis is risk assessment. Scientific risk assessment is the process of determining the relation between exposure to a hazard at a specific magnitude and the likelihood of an adverse event or disease (IOM, 1997). The science should characterize the nature and magnitude of risks to human health associated with food related hazards. On the basis of the scientific assessment, regulators can make informed decisions about where and how to allocate resources to prevent and control hazards. The same scientific technique can sometimes be used for a range of problems throughout the entire system. Uniformity in the process of risk measurement can reduce uncertainty about how specific foods or processes will be addressed, and thus benefit non-regulatory components of the system as well.

Adequate Surveillance and Monitoring

Strong surveillance and technical support provide an infrastructure to set priorities for research, education, and response. Food safety, perhaps more than any other health-related activity of government, demands a continuing and dynamic "moving picture" of the system, rather than periodic "snapshots." For successful leadership, the federal system requires the ability to identify and set priorities among potential food safety hazards and emerging issues. Surveillance and monitoring, education and research, and enforcement and regulation are all used to identify, set priorities among, and address concerns.

Surveillance is the first step toward building the capacity to detect and respond to sporadic instances and outbreaks of foodborne illness. Surveillance and monitoring are also essential for evaluating the system, identifying emerging issues and new trends, and assessing risk from the farm or sea to the table. Monitoring foodborne disease and related hazards can allow early and rapid detection of hazards and illnesses. Thorough investigation of outbreaks to determine their sources and causes can identify crucial weaknesses in the system.

Focused Education and Research

Part of the role of the federal government in ensuring safe food is to promote education and research. Continuous, high-quality research is needed to keep capabilities of regulators up-to-date and to ensure rational and maximally effective evaluation and decision-making as well as optimal preventive measures.

Effective education, the strongest and most important form of information transfer, requires partnerships at the federal, state, regional, and local levels. The federal government should lead efforts to educate and inform the general public on such issues as labeling (including health and nutrition information), standards and specifications, changing technologies, and advertising. All stakeholders in the food system should be fully informed of risks and of food-handling practices that reduce those risks.

Both the responsibilities and the needs for setting education and outreach priorities are shared among many stakeholders. Integration and collaboration can help to focus efforts where the needs are greatest. Priorities for education are closely tied to communication capabilities and should be based on need. General academic and land-grant institutions in partnership with private industry and a variety of organizations play critical roles in the transfer of information. Producers, processors, and consumers have needs for both general and specialized education.

Carefully planned education programs to communicate fundamental issues are important, with additional opportunities for education in times of crisis. Both should be used during major or highly publicized foodborne illness events. Education about the critical role of consumers in the food safety system might be especially effective.

Research priorities should be focused on the prevention of foodborne illness; this requires research on measures of current problems to determine how the problems can best be brought under control. Specifically, research priorities should be related closely to needs as determined by effective surveillance.

Some research priorities in an effective food safety system must be responsive to emerging problems, but others must have a long-term perspective, and effective research management requires a capability to shift resources and emphasis. In the past, research priorities have often been based on opportunities or pressing issues of the moment. Typically, research funding has been event-driven, rather than evenly sustained in support of longer-term objectives. The press of current problems is an ever-present threat to the needed long-range research, and an effective food safety system will support and protect both. Research must always be relevant to societal concerns and to the complex problems of ensuring a safe food supply. Research priorities should be established internally and externally in partnership with private industry, academe, consumers, and other stakeholders. The priorities must be widely known and accepted; it can be difficult for any agency to maintain an appropriate long-term balance when the news media, the public, legislators, and others, direct issues to be set aside when a crises of the moment arises.

The research budget, especially for long-term projects, should be protected from rapid swings and decreases. Perhaps more than most other activities, the development of effective research teams requires development over time, with significant effort, patience, and resources. A single lean budget can destroy the benefits of effective team-building efforts over a period of many years.

Not every research need can be met, but a force of the best scientific research investigators are needed to solve the long-term, difficult, and highly complex issues of food safety. These experts must be dedicated to the mission of protecting public health by ensuring a safe food supply and they must not be distracted by needs for research in other fields, such as improved methods of food production or processing, or treatment of food related illnesses.

Effective and Consistent Regulation and Enforcement

Mechanisms for the prevention of foodborne illness can span the spectrum from voluntary to regulatory and from outright bans to warning labels and education. Regulation is often intended to be a preventive and protective measure. A prerequisite for any regulatory action should be the assurance of adequate, consistent, and effective enforcement. The ability to protect requires the authority and resources to take action. The food safety system must contain adequate provisions for enforcement of regulations and must clearly link responsibilities with accountabilities. Many challenges posed by the current food safety structure, as described in Chapter five of this report, result from an inability to take action, respond to needs, or protect.

Consistency is important in all aspects of ensuring safe food. Similar risks require similar planning, actions, and response. For instance, the intensity, nature, and frequency of inspection should be consistent for foods associated with like risks.

Response and Adaptation to New Technology and Changing Consumer Needs

The food supply and food production, processing, distribution and consumption practices in the United States have changed dramatically during the past 70 years. Further major changes will certainly occur, though it cannot be predicted when or what they will be. The fundamental shifts from a few, largely local items to today's variety, from small neighborhood stores to supermarkets, from familiar individual ingredients to prepared foods, from home to outside preparation or consumption, and from traditional to "ethnic" cuisine were not widely predicted before they were well in progress. As these shifts continue to occur, the technologies associated with production, processing, manufacturing, and delivery of food also continue to change.

Hazards associated with food consumption also are continually changing. In recent years, the risks associated with fresh fruits and vegetables have grown because of increased consumption, variety, and importation of produce from developing countries (GAO, 1998). Importation of different types and amounts of foods from outside the United States expands the federal responsibilities and expertise needed in the US food safety system.

The system must include primary prevention of new food hazards through research and other activities and be flexible to respond to new and potential hazards. The food revolutions of this century have proceeded irregularly and often simultaneously, but few have been adequately anticipated. It is certain that revolution will continue, and an effective food safety system will prepare for the known as well as for future hazards that cannot be clearly seen.

The changing attitudes, concerns, desires, needs, and roles of consumers dictate the characteristics of the food supply and its associated risks. The United States has become home to people of many origins and cultures. With those cultures has come the desire for particular foods. A great challenge to a food safety system is to meet the changing demands while securing safety of a rapidly expanding and diversifying food supply.

Human and Financial Resources

The immense responsibility of an effective food safety system is coupled with the need for adequate human and financial support. If federal and other programs are to prevent, identify, track, control, and respond to food related illness and reduce risks of future outbreaks or hazards, they will require commensurate funding. Insufficient funding and lack of incentives can diminish an ability to inspect and control foodborne illness; curtail needed research; prevent sustainable, aggressive, and innovative education efforts; and create instability in the system. For instance, the role of states as a public partner in the food safety system has traditionally been important. State and local regulators can help to ensure the safety of food in commerce, and they can assume responsibility for monitoring and enforcing safe food-handling practices; but adequate state and federal funding is needed to carry out these tasks.

The economic costs and benefits of reducing the risk of foodborne illness are difficult to determine accurately and consistently. Regulations that govern the production, processing, distribution, and marketing of food can create benefits by improving food safety, but they can also increase producers' costs and potentially raise food prices. The economic costs of inaction are difficult to assess because the data typically reflect only reported incidents and deaths; unreported events generally elude economic assessment. Net benefits of increasing food safety can be maximized by equating the marginal benefits of safer food with the marginal costs of achieving food safety goals. Market-oriented approaches to food safety include economic incentives. In addition, personnel must be trained, developed, and kept up-to-date with advances and innovations elsewhere. Scientific and managerial competence must be ensured to build the human capacity necessary to support the system.

Provision of adequate funding and staffing are not sufficient; the system must also be efficient and cost-effective. One cost-effective measure is early detection and early warning of outbreaks before they spread. Federal coordination with regard to research and education efforts can ensure rapid and efficient response.

Every system should be practical. The mission must be practical, the goals must be attainable, and the work must be feasible. Primary food hazard prevention approaches and research (both long-term and short-term) efforts must focus on practical applications. Inspection, surveillance and monitoring, and education programs should be practical in their gathering and conveying of information.

The federal government plays a prominent role in ensuring that vital elements are in place and that the unifying mission of food safety is sufficiently addressed. The coordinated application of scientific, technical, and regulatory measures to prevent foodborne illness and promote public health and safety is critical to the federal government's mission, with its core responsibility to ensure an effective food safety system. There are also occasions where regulatory activity can encourage or require the use of new technologies, which causes movement toward higher standards in the system.

THE ROLES OF PRIVATE SECTOR PARTNERS

Private partners working in an effective food safety system include producers and importers, processors, marketers (retail and wholesale), food services, trade organizations, professional societies, and private organizations.

The primary and common roles of the various private-sector partners include bringing food to the tables of consumers and bringing sound scientific information to others in the partnership. Within the food production system, the private sector has the primary responsibility for ensuring food safety. To be most effective in this task, the private sector must maintain close interaction with the public sector, which sets standards and provides oversight, and with the consuming public, which expresses its food needs and choices. Many of the important attributes of an effective food safety system are included in a recent report, *Guiding Principles for Optimum Food Safety Oversight and Regulation in the United States,* endorsed by 13 professional, scientific societies (IFT, 1998).

The roles and contributions of specific private partners are varied and distinctive, and each can make unique contributions to the overall functioning of an effective system. Several examples of successful partnerships that highlight private roles in the framework of an effective food safety system are provided below.

Producers

Production in some areas may represent the least controlled point in the food supply system. However, there are valuable opportunities for effective partnerships between producers and governments in the food safety system. An example of a combination of regulatory and non-regulatory partnership between producers and federal and state governments is the National Poultry Improvement Plan (NPIP), in which state authorities cooperate with the US

Department of Agriculture to administer regulations for the improvement of poultry, poultry products, and hatcheries.

In this example, industry participants follow both the general provisions of the plan and specific provisions that are related to their industry category—hatcheries, dealers, and breeders. Food animal industries use and understand on-farm quality assurance or control programs; these could be expanded to include food safety provisions if they are cost-effective and serve as an incentive to market products. The industries are to follow all sanitary provisions and undergo testing and inspection. The industries pay most costs of the plan and seek to achieve and maintain a free or "clean" status. The plan has been useful, especially in breeding flocks, and has helped to eliminate several poultry diseases and prevent the spread of disease from breeders to commercial flocks. More recently, the NPIP adapted an on-farm sanitation program to prevent and control the serious human pathogen *Salmonella enteritidis* in hatching eggs and chicks.

The NPIP provides a working model that involves federal-state-industry partnership. Industry members use the findings to inform the public that they have met the highest standards and have free, or "clean," status, a designation that adds value to their products and is a "preharvest" animal-production model that might be used in an expanded version for other food animal species. Federal and state agencies benefit from reduced requirements for inspection and oversight of "clean" facilities.

Processors, Marketers, and Distributors

The dairy processing industry recognized the need for effective control of foodborne pathogens by promoting the enactment of effective controls of milkborne disease, including pasteurization. To assist states and municipalities in their efforts to prevent milkborne disease, the US Public Health Service developed model regulations for voluntary adoption by state and local milk-control agencies in 1924. A model milk regulation, the Grade A Pasteurized Milk Ordinance, was developed and implemented through partnerships between the dairy industry and federal, state, and local regulatory agencies.

Private industry can contribute to the shaping of the scientific basis of the future food safety system. For example, the Flavor and Extract Manufacturers Association (FEMA) and the Food and Drug Administration (FDA) developed the FEMA Generally Recognized as Safe review program to ensure the safety of food flavors and extracts. In another example of industry-FDA cooperation, the development of low-acid, canned food regulations was a major step toward the safety of canned foods by reducing risks of botulism. Those examples illustrate how a progressive, scientific partnership can contribute to a food safety system.

Education and information transfer can also be important contributions of private industry and its associated trade organizations. For instance, the Food Distributors International and its retail partners have engaged in a cooperative food safety initiative, implemented through the Food Marketing Institute. This project assists the allied food industries to share information, to keep up to date on regulatory developments and technical resources in food safety, and to develop and maintain procedures for the industry.

The egg industry has integrated government efforts, academic research, and other industries to address food safety concerns. The industry has implemented new technologies developed by government and academe to reduce foodborne illness, has developed model partnerships, and has educated and informed consumers about the safety and nutritional composition of egg products.

THE ROLE OF THE CONSUMER

Consumers have a large and critical role in an effective food safety system. First, the food system revolves around the purchasing power and decisions of consumers. Annual expenditures for food are enormous—over $700 billion in the United States (Putnam and Allshouse, 1997). More important, the health, well-being, and longevity of the nation's population ultimately depend on individual consumer decisions. As discussed earlier, it is the role of the private (industrial) sector to deliver to consumers food that is wholesome and safe and food that can be rendered or maintained safe by appropriate handling and preparation by the consumer. After food leaves the production and distribution systems, a different set of risks affects food that is prepared and consumed at home, for which only consumers can be responsible for safety, and food that is prepared by commercial establishments away from home (restaurants, takeout shops, grocery store delicatessens), for which vendors retain major responsibilities for safety, although consumers must still follow good safety practices.

As has been noted before, the food system and the food safety system have constantly changed in many ways to meet consumers' perceived needs. This evolution has depended on close interactions between government and the private sector, but the role of government is often unseen except during crisis situations. Continuing activities of the government and the private sector provide the foundation of a safe food supply, but they must also provide the information and education that consumers need if they are to meet their own responsibilities.

Although consumers' desires, needs, and cultures have changed, the basic standards of food hygiene in the home have changed very little and probably will not change much in the foreseeable future (See Box 4-2). The food safety system should continue to include fundamental information about frequent and effective washing, prompt refrigeration, and proper cooling. Consumer knowledge on good practices is essential to consumer action, including handling, storage, and preparation of food in ways that improve food safety. Consumers should have reason for confidence that food and food components are safe when received, and they should know how to protect their food as it moves through preparation and consumption.

The size and importance of the consumer interactions with the food system have contributed to the growth of consumer organizations. These play an important role, particularly in advocacy about food safety matters. In addition, they help greatly by providing education and information. They should be involved in the development of protocols and studies to fill the vital information needs of the food safety system. Their leadership role requires them to ensure that their positions on food safety issues are science-based, and that they fairly represent the concerns of consumers in their advocacy role.

BOX 4-2   The Consumer's Role in Food Safety

In the early 1900s, pasteurization of milk was becoming common. It was the consumer's responsibility to preserve the quality of milk after it was delivered to the home. The consumer was instructed that "as soon as possible after the milk is set on the doorstep, it should be taken in and put in a cold part of the ice box. If some time must elapse between delivery and care by the consumer, an insulated box should be provided to protect the milk from heat and/or freezing. Milk should be placed only in clean pitchers or receptacles. Milk that has stood at room temperature during a meal should not be poured back into cold, fresh milk, but kept in its own container." Keep clean and cold was the rule that was followed to preserve the quality and flavor of milk.

Today, the rule of almost a century ago still applies to consumer responsibility, as is demonstrated by the Fight BAC campaign's educational message. New mechanisms for production, processing, and delivery have evolved, but consumers remain responsible for ensuring that milk and other products are kept clean and cold. (USDA, 1939; Partnership for Food Safety Education, 1997b).

THE ROLE OF OTHER PARTNERS

Government, the private sector, and consumers are not the only recognized organizations that are vitally involved in the food safety system. Scientists, educators, and food specialists are also key partners who are placed throughout the system and in academic institutions. For example, the Institute of Food Technologists represents food scientists, and the American Veterinary Medical Association represents veterinarians in industry, academe, and government agencies. Both professional organizations have subgroups that interact with the government agencies.

The news media cannot be considered an active partner in a food safety system, but are important players. Objective, accurate reporting about food hazards and timely transfer of information to the general public are essential.

The news media also engage in efforts to educate the public about basic food hygiene.

In an effective food safety system these groups are recognized for their distinct and important roles and are encouraged to participate by membership on advisory groups, by providing direct input to the regulatory process, or by other actions.

A DYNAMIC INTERDEPENDENCE

Ensuring safe food is an appropriate role for government, but that role is not exclusive, nor is it a contract between government and the American public to guarantee absolute safety. A strong government presence may be necessary for a strong food safety system but is not necessarily sufficient to create a stronger and better food safety system. An effective food safety system is based on a particular set of attributes and relationships and a focus on improving the public's health and well-being, and the roles of federal, state, and local governments must be well defined, coordinated, and consistent in achieving a single mission.

The public often turns its attention to what government *should* do rather than what government *can* do. But what can government at its various levels actually do to promote food safety, and what conditions must exist to optimize its performance? The answers to those questions are based on defining the functions of the food safety system that can best be performed by each of the actors and on the ability to fill in system gaps in light of the inherent limitations of public service today. What can others or other systems do just as well or better, and should they? An effective food safety system is built on fusing the strengths of multiple players, by linking roles and authorities to responsibilities, and by aligning shareholders' efforts toward a single overarching mission of public health. An effective system emphasizes partnerships new and old, integration, and the need for accountability of all participants.

The food safety system in the twenty-first century should be based on a framework of common goals, measures, rewards, teams, and networks that focus on outcomes. Once the framework is developed and operating to address desired outcomes, and once the attributes of a successful system have been integrated, optimum features of a final organizational design will be more apparent. There is a critical need to connect the food system strategically with an effective food safety component; this cannot be an afterthought but rather must be a planned and purposeful activity.

It is clear that the food safety system must function as a integrated enterprise. That is, it must be agile, fluid, connected, integrated, and transparent. Integration is the antithesis of a system with components in isolation, barriers, and disconnected functions, rules, and policies. One of the most important aspects of an effective food safety system is the ability to assume an active, preventive role, as opposed to a reactive mode, to deal with problems already present. Focusing on prevention of foodborne illness rather than on response to failures is key to identifying and controlling outbreaks of foodborne illness. The system must be built to resolve today's problems but also with a special contemplation and flexibility to address future needs that are not yet foreseeable in detail.

Most important, systems for continuous improvement must be based on information and science. Feedback processes are critical to learning, improvement, and change. The food system requires good data at numerous points to measure results and adapt processes.

A unified food safety mission implies that goals are adopted to protect the public health, reduce risks of foodborne illness, and maintain, build, or rebuild consumer confidence. Means for evaluation and feedback are needed to determine whether the food safety system is meeting its goals. The criteria for assessment of the system outcomes include verifiable measures of progress, such as reduced numbers of foodborne illness outbreaks, decreased incidence of chemical residues in food, and a better understanding of foodborne risks that improves public policy and promotes improved consumer practices.

SUMMARY FINDINGS: An Effective Food Safety System

- Should be science-based with a strong emphasis on risk analysis and prevention, thus allowing the greatest priority in terms of resources and activity to be placed on the risks deemed to have the greatest potential impact;
- is based on a national food law that is clear, rational, and scientifically based on risk;
- includes comprehensive surveillance and monitoring activities which serve as a basis for risk analysis;
- has one central voice at the federal level which is responsible for food safety and has the authority and resources to implement science-based policy in all federal activities related to food safety;
- recognizes the responsibilities and central role played by the nonfederal partners (state, local, industry, consumers) in the food safety system; and
- receives adequate funding to carry out major functions required.

5

Where Current US Food Safety Activities Fall Short

Over three decades ago, Thomas Kuhn suggested that scientific paradigms remain dominant until they fail to solve new problems (Kuhn, 1962). As the burden of unsolved problems grows, ultimately a new paradigm arises and focuses major shifts in thinking and even changes in institutions. While a new paradigm works well at first, it is likely to work less and less well over time until a new paradigm is needed. This model describes our food safety system today.

The recognition that foodborne illnesses and deaths cost this country billions of dollars a year coincides with an apparent lack of public trust in government and gives rise to the suggestion that government is the problem, not a solution. That is a disconcerting depiction and, in one important respect, it is inaccurate. Officials who direct or carry out diverse functions under the multiplicity of statutory mandates are capable and dedicated, as are their state and local counterparts. They perform remarkably well, given their budgetary and statutory constraints, but they operate within an institutional framework that is out of date and poorly designed to accomplish the critical goals that regulation in this field must achieve. The increasing complexity of food production and delivery and the exploding internationalization of the US food supply impose added pressure on the federal regulatory apparatus which was constructed in simpler times.

Given the challenges, the US food safety system has several strengths. Problems are addressed at many points from production to consumption and from many different perspectives (for example, federal or state, public or private, top-down or investigator-initiated, basic or applied, and combined or separated from regulatory pressures). There are significant efforts to improve the current structure through implementation of systems with multiple critical control points to address hazards and increase safety. There is a shared sense of urgency and commitment arising from the current national emphasis on food safety which has resulted in extensive communication and coordination efforts throughout the system (interagency, agency and industry, and state and federal).

79

There is also substantial private funding in support of food safety research. In spite of these strengths, the current food safety system that the committee studied displays several fundamental weaknesses, which are described on the following pages.

INADEQUATE APPLICATION OF SCIENCE

Rapid changes in the US food system and spectacular recent scientific advances have only slowly affected food safety policies and regulations. The US Department of Agriculture (USDA), the Food and Drug Administration (FDA), the Environmental Protection Agency (EPA), and the National Institutes of Health (NIH) will collectively spend an estimated $170.8 million on food safety research in 1998 (Appendix E), but there is minimal coordination and little integration of their efforts. The absence of a nationally coordinated research agenda for food safety raises serious concerns about duplication of effort and about the linkage of science to attempt to solve food safety problems of the highest priority.

In some federal departments, such as the USDA, authorities for research and regulation are separated and assigned to different agencies. In other agencies, such as the FDA and the EPA, the regulatory agencies also have authority for research. Separation of research from the constantly changing pressures and priorities of the regulatory environment facilitates science-driven research that requires long-term commitments. The separation is also appropriate for research targeted principally at producers, processors, educators, consumers, and non-regulatory scientists. But combining research and regulation in the same agency facilitates implementation of the research and improves focus on the highest-priority regulatory needs. Such a combination also strengthens the science and technology base of the regulatory agency. However, in spite of growing national concern about foodborne illnesses, both research and its scientific base for the regulatory programs in the FDA were slowly eroding prior to the *Food Safety from Farm to Table: A National Food-Safety Initiative* (Appendix C); this trend appears to be changing with the current actual and proposed increased funding for food safety research (Appendix E).

Both rapid scientific response and long-term research are needed to adequately address food safety issues. Although USDA's Agricultural Research Service (ARS) has the organizational structure to respond quickly, it might not have the scientific expertise or other resources required for a specific research need of USDA's Food Safety and Inspection Service (FSIS). It might not be willing (or in some instances authorized) to redirect resources to an FSIS need if redirection would disrupt its long-term research programs. In short, ARS does not meet all the research needs of FSIS. FSIS is working with other agencies (USDA's Cooperative State Research, Education and Extension Service [CSREES], NIH, and FDA) to persuade them to target more of their research programs specifically to the FSIS agenda. Communication and coordination of the CSREES research agenda with FSIS does not appear to be well-developed even though both agencies are in the same department.

RESEARCH FUNDING LEVELS

The committee conducted a public forum in which spokespersons representing several industry and consumer groups cited the need for adequate federal funding of food safety research, and two former FSIS administrators emphasized the need for increased research funding throughout the federal system (Appendix D). President Clinton's fiscal year 1999 budget proposes increased funding for food safety research as part of the National Food Safety Initiative. There is value in having research programs, some of which are responsive to regulatory activities and some to longer term or differently targeted research programs, protected from short-term regulatory pressures. The nation needs epidemiological research on human pathogens on the farm, but the attempts of FSIS to obtain this information are limited by statutory and funding restrictions. Other agencies can do even less at the producer level. Concerns about the adequacy of research funding can be further exemplified by a broader consideration of the issue.

Most federal research efforts directed toward human-pathogen control at the farm-level are in ARS. In 1997, ARS had 18 research projects involving 51 scientists (excluding graduate and postdoctoral students) who were committed to the control of foodborne pathogens in live animals (Panter and Robens, 1997). The recent development of a product to reduce *Salmonella enteritidis* in chickens (Macriowski et al., 1997) indicates the scientific quality and relevance of that program. However, in the judgment of the committee, the scale and scope of the ARS program are not commensurate with the urgency of the problem, the potential impact of the preharvest approach, or the knowledge gap and scientific complexity of the issues. Understanding the epidemiology, ecology, and molecular mechanisms involved in the array of pathogens confronted and the control procedures needed at the farm level require a larger investment. Funding for extramural programs is not adequate to fill the gap. For example, the total CSREES funding for all food safety research at the 115 extramural institutions participating in CSREES food safety research programs in Fiscal Year 1998 is $9.9 million (Appendix E). Even though those funds are leveraged by state and private investments, they fall far short of the funding required for optimal use of the research resources of the participating institutions in solving the nation's food safety problems. A 1994 National Research Council report emphasizes the need for increased funding of food safety research through the CSREES (NRC, 1994). The relatively modest increases in CSREES funding for food safety research in the last two years were greatly needed but are not adequate for national needs.

Recent Efforts to Improve Research

In an effort to address a portion of the scientific inadequacies of the system, the President directed the Secretaries of the Department of Health and Human Services and the USDA to create a Joint Institute for Food Safety Research that would: (1) develop a strategic plan for conducting food safety research activities consistent with the National Food-Safety Initiative; and (2) efficiently coordinate all federal food safety research, including research conducted with the private sector and academe (Office of the President, 1998). The principal goals of this joint institute is to develop the means to identify foodborne hazards more rapidly and accurately, and to develop effective interventions to prevent food contamination at each step from farm to table. While these actions are significant steps toward improving food safety research, there remain major shortfalls in the application of science in the current system, which include:

- There is no nationally coordinated scientific research agenda among all agencies involved in food safety that stems from a unified mission or centrally focused leadership.
- There is a lack of adequate integration of research efforts among agencies.
- Resources currently identified for research are inadequate to support a science-based system.

INADEQUATE USE OF RISK ASSESSMENT

It is widely recognized that eating food entails an inherent risk of illness. The risk of acquiring foodborne illness can vary widely and depends on the type of food and how the food is processed, handled, and prepared. Some foods, such as commercial sterile, retorted canned products, present a very low risk of transmitting foodborne pathogens; others, such as raw oysters, have a well-documented history of disseminating foodborne disease.

Risk assessment determines the probability of illness caused by eating food contaminated with specific foodborne hazards. Critical information needed for risk assessment includes identification of the hazardous agent, data on the prevalence and concentrations of the agent in specific foods, profiles of the consumption of specific foods, and the disease response of people who are exposed to different amounts of the harmful agent. Those data are used in a mathematical calculation to estimate the risk of illness to a specific category of consumers that is caused by a harmful agent in a specific type of food. However, quantitative microbial risk assessment is a new discipline that is in the developmental stages, and refinements are needed before it can be fully implemented.

The limited availability of resources to address food safety issues necessitates that priorities among safety programs be set on the basis of risk assessment. That approach to assessing the relative safety of different foods enables regulators to estimate the probability of acquiring illness from eating specific foods and thereby allows them to place the greatest emphasis on foods that have the highest risk of causing human illness. Hence, risk assessment is a science-based approach to addressing food safety issues. It is not, however, to be restrictive; dealing with several small risks may be more effective and less expensive than efforts to eliminate a large but intractable problem.

The major shortfall with regard to the use of risk assessment in the current system includes:

- Under the current statutory and budgetary constraints, it is not possible to fully realize the benefits of the valuable and critical tool of risk assessment and its resulting positive impacts on food safety.

INSUFFICIENT INFORMATION

A glaring weakness of the current US food safety system is a lack of information. This gap impedes our identification, description, and elimination of problems. There is a lack of knowledge about the seriousness, incidence, and cost of foodborne disease. There is inadequate information on the type of foods that people eat in various regions of the United States, the size of portions, how they are prepared, and how often they are eaten. Information is lacking on the association of pathogens with food animals, and on the prevalence of chemical and physical hazards. Methods and critical control points for reducing or eliminating pathogens in different parts of the food system, especially in production, are insufficient.

The paucity of information to link key players in the food system results in few feedback systems for continuous evaluation and improvement. For instance, mechanisms are lacking for tracing a diseased animal back to point of production on the farm; this impedes objective assessment of the current situation and prevents the ability to reduce the likelihood of future incidents. The committee could not assess with confidence the severity and impact of on-farm food-related hazards, because the risk could not be quantified. This lack of information also impedes the direction of new efforts and the measurement of progress associated with changes in private-sector conduct or government policy.

Current understanding of the magnitude of the problem of foodborne disease and the relative importance of the relevant hazards is inadequate and in many cases inaccurate. Furthermore, the scientific resources and structure are lacking to address the inadequacies and inaccuracies. Effective and adequate monitoring, surveillance, and research to characterize risk are required to improve the allocation of resources and to develop the knowledge and technology needed to manage hazards that pose the greatest risk.

The major shortfall regarding available information in the current system can be summarized as:

- There is a serious lack of information to allow appropriate characterization, assessment, and response to the problem of foodborne hazards in the United States.

HACCP SYSTEMS AND THEIR LIMITATIONS

Federal food safety agencies are shifting to a new conceptual framework based on hazard identification and process control—the science-based Hazard Analysis Critical Control Point (HACCP) program for the prevention of pathogen dissemination. However, for this program to be successful, government must find new ways to deploy its financial and personnel resources. There is serious concern about the lack of sufficient resources for USDA to provide timely implementation of HACCP-based inspection in processing facilities. Most federal inspection resources are committed by statute to carcass-by-carcass inspection of meat and poultry. Current resources are not adequate to meet statutory requirements and to train and hire the federal regulatory personnel required to implement HACCP programs fully throughout the food safety system.

Implementation of HACCP systems throughout the food continuum is a major step toward enhancing food safety, but HACCP systems should not be thought of as preventing all human illnesses resulting from consumption of potentially hazardous foods. Some potentially hazardous foods are produced and processed with HACCP systems that do not involve a treatment that will kill pathogens. The control points used in processing foods like fresh meat and poultry might not kill harmful bacteria, such as *Salmonella*, but only prevent their growth; refrigeration could be an example of such a control point. Foods with pathogens that have been controlled or reduced, but not eliminated, could still cause human illness. Hence, although HACCP systems properly implemented throughout the food continuum should greatly reduce the incidence of foodborne illnesses, vehicles for contamination and disease may still remain.

The major shortfalls regarding HACCP systems include:

- Under current statutory and budgetary constraints, the benefits of HACCP systems in enhancing the safety of foods cannot be fully realized.
- HACCP systems can minimize risk but cannot assure absolute safety of potentially hazardous foods that do not receive a treatment to destroy harmful microorganisms.

ABSENCE OF FOCUSED LEADERSHIP

No single federal official can be said to be responsible for the government's food safety efforts. Instead, several officials have responsibility for parts of the system that are organizationally separate and individually funded. Many of the separate programs have other responsibilities as well. They are in different parts of the executive branch and they report to different congressional oversight and appropriation committees. Sometimes they compete for resources and for public attention. None of the heads of these agencies has direct access to the White House, and several report through more than one administrative level. *Food Safety from Farm to Table: A National Food Safety Initiative* (Appendix C) has given more prominence to the federal government's role generally, but it has not fundamentally or permanently altered the underlying balkanized structure.

Fulfillment of the federal role in protecting the food supply requires central management of now-dispersed efforts. Central management is essential if resources are to be allocated in accord with science-based assessments of risk and potential benefit. It is necessary to assume cooperation among dispersed, sometimes competing, programs. It is important for coordination among the states and between the states and localities and the federal government. It is also the only way to ensure that a focused federal entity is responsible for food safety policy.

The major shortfalls regarding leadership in the current system include:

- There is no single federal entity that is both responsible for the government's efforts and that has the authority to implement policy and designate resources toward food safety activities.
- There is a lack of a unified mission among the various agencies with regard to food safety.

STATUTORY LIMITATIONS

There is no "food safety" counterpart of such modern federal regulatory laws as the Clean Air Act or the Occupational Safety and Health Act, and there is no comparable legal framework for federal food safety activities. Primary authority for food safety is bifurcated between the USDA and the FDA, and other responsibilities are more widely dispersed. There is no formal structure for coordinating or empowering state regulatory bodies (which in many states are themselves divided along USDA-FDA lines). Federal support for and administration of relevant scientific research are even more widely dispersed and uncoordinated.

Some of the numerous reasons for this state of affairs are obvious. The most important date from the beginning of the century, when Congress made two choices that decisively influence federal regulation to this day. First, it assigned responsibility for ensuring the safety of meat to one agency and responsibility for other foods to another. That division of authority would have impeded coherent federal regulation even if the threats to food safety had remained unchanged. But they have not remained unchanged, and the result has been to make unmistakably clear the misallocation of regulatory effort that is the product of Congress' second critical decision—its current directive, embedded in statute, that each meat (and later poultry) carcass must be subject to physical inspection. That decision although it may have been appropriate for the hazards present 70 years ago, impedes FSIS efforts to allocate its substantial regulatory resources in ways that correspond to the health risks presented by contemporary sources of food or modern means of food production and processing. In short, the hazards of greatest concern today are microbiological and chemical contamination; and they are not detectable with the traditional inspection by look, sound, smell, and feel. The law's demand has for decades influenced funding of meat and poultry regulation.

The statutory structure impedes coherent, risk-based regulation in other ways. The responsibilities given to FDA emphasize control of the use of chemicals in food production and the addition of chemicals to food. The relevant post-World War II amendments to the Federal Food, Drug, and Cosmetic Act (FDCA) have addressed that apparent threat for conventional foods. The provisions of the FDCA that address food sanitation remain as they were passed 60 years ago, when lawmakers concluded that poor food sanitation poses greater threats.

The discrepancy between regulatory effort and risk is increased because of the way the law's requirements are implemented. Generally speaking, any chemical proposed to be added to food or used in food production must have agency approval before it can be used, unless it is an ingredient in a dietary supplement. The law obligates FDA or EPA to entertain and rule promptly on applications for new food additives. Although the agencies rarely meet statutory deadlines, their legal obligations to rule on new chemicals have led them—and Congress—to allocate major resources to this function and to neglect activities directed toward food sanitation.

Passage of the 1994 Dietary Supplement Health and Education Act provided for the sale of dietary supplements that do not present a significant or unreasonable risk of illness when used as recommended on the label or under ordinary conditions of use. Some consumers believe that if a small amount of these supplements is beneficial, then more will be more beneficial; this poses the risk of adverse health effects due to overconsumption. Current law makes consumer protection against any potential risk difficult.

Neither the Meat Products Inspection Act nor the Poultry Products Inspection Act speaks to how livestock are produced, maintained, or managed. FDA and EPA, respectively, prescribe conditions for food use of animal drugs and feed additives and for pesticides. These conditions are meant to prevent the presence of dangerous amounts of those chemicals in food. However, monitoring of compliance with approved usage is poorly funded and episodic.

State and local authorities have more to say about on-farm practices, but their monitoring capabilities are severely limited.

Most food processors operate in interstate commerce and therefore are subject to FDA standards and inspection. But, as has been noted, the FDCA does not require food processors to register with the agency, so FDA's knowledge of its universe is incomplete.

FDA's shrunken inspection force is seriously over-extended, and FDA appears to have insufficient resources to meet its statutory obligations. For example, numbers of FDA food inspections are declining: premises regulated by The Center for Food Safety and Applied Nutrition are inspected on the average once every 10 years (GAO, 1994b). New technologies, products, and processes continue to need timely regulatory review and decision. As technical people retire or leave the agency, resources must be adequate to attract highly qualified people to fill these public service roles. User fees have been suggested and rejected as a fiscal solution. In the meantime, such reform efforts as the FDA Modernization Act of 1997 increase FDA's workload, at least for the near term. Congress must provide appropriate resources for the tasks demanded of FDA.

Another growing segment of the food industry largely escapes federal oversight: food service establishments—including full-service restaurants, fast-food establishments, grocery store delicatessens, and sidewalk food vendors—whose sales together now account for over 45 percent of the American food dollar (Putnam and Allshouse, 1997). The materials and ingredients that the establishments purchase are theoretically subject to federal regulation, but their food preparation activities are not. It is a matter of debate whether federal law potentially applies to these activities, but it is clear that federal officials leave regulation of them to the states and localities, where monitoring and enforcement are vulnerable to budgetary pressures, jurisdictional disputes, and diverse legal standards.

The major statutory shortfall of the current system is that:

- There are inconsistent, uneven, and at times archaic food statutes that inhibit use of science-based decision-making in activities related to food safety, and these statutes can be inconsistently interpreted and enforced among agencies.

LACK OF COORDINATION

A lack of coordination on several levels seems to be one effect of the lack of strong focused leadership and the lack of a unified mission. The lack of coordination has resulted in a lack of national standards and a lack of focus on food safety. There appear to be no mechanisms to sustain expanding interagency coordination after the current national concern abates and the attention of Congress, the President, and agency leadership is directed to other issues.

Several examples of coordination deficiencies include:

Lack of federal agency coordination. Surveillance information is ultimately communicated among the agencies and organizations involved, but there is (except for the recent creation of FoodNet) no integration of the various programs included in the current structure. Neither routine surveillance programs, special projects, nor emerging issues are addressed in a coordinated interagency manner. There is no comprehensive national strategy or system for surveillance. Human and animal studies and analyses of foods are, for the most part, conducted independently without a common goal or design, even though they may impact the same food safety issues.

Another example is the lack of coordination between FDA and USDA regarding the regulation and clearance of packaging materials. For instance, catalyst systems used to make polymers do not appear in the FDA food additive regulations because they are understood to be proprietary information. However, USDA now requires companies to file a food additive petition with FDA for catalyst systems.

Lack of federal and state coordination. Federal, state, and local authorities must work with varied amounts of resources, skills, and legal authority. Lack of coordination and consistency between federal and state governments is problematic. Some states have initiatives requiring more stringent standards than those required by the federal government. Under California's Proposition 65, warnings may be required for products, including foods, that are not required under federal law. Another example of a lack of federal and state coordination is that food retailers with stores in multiple states must deal with many regulatory entities at the federal, state, and local levels. The committee heard testimony from the Food Marketing Institute (FMI) indicating that one food retailer with stores in several states must report to 88 different regulatory authorities. (Jill Hollingsworth, FMI, personal communication to committee, April 1998; Appendix D). These conflicting requirements create an additional burden on industry and may confuse consumers.

Lack of public and private coordination. As described by the United Food and Commercial Workers Union, implementation of HACCP programs in meat packing plants is often required and attempted without allowing time to perform proper cleaning or to conduct effective employee training (Jackie Nowell, United Food and Commercial Workers Union, personal communication to committee, April 1998; Appendix D).

Lack of international coordination. Currently, sampling of imported foods takes place at the port-of-entry (GAO, 1998). This method of inspection does not allow for the timely identification of potential foodborne hazards. There is a need to identify and correct problems at the point where food is produced and processed, and this requires international government coordination and cooperation.

The major shortfalls regarding coordination in the current system include:

- There is a lack of coordination and integration among the at least 12 agencies that are involved in implementing the 35 primary statues that regulate food safety.
- There is often ineffective or insufficient coordination among federal, state, local, and private entities.

DEFICIENCIES IN REGULATION OF IMPORTED FOOD

Protecting the safety of domestically produced food is a daunting challenge, but the country's growing reliance on imported food adds several layers of complexity. It is by no means clear that imported food, as a class, poses greater risks than does domestically produced food. What is clear is that federal officials cannot use the same methods in regulating imported food that they use—or that would make sense—in regulating domestically produced food. Methods that rely on production-site monitoring of compliance with safety standards or universal physical inspection of marketed shipments cannot be directly translated overseas.

The laws that FSIS and FDA administer require that imported food meet the same standards as domestic food. But the enforcement approaches of the two agencies to meet this common requirement are quite different. FSIS statutory authority requires meat and poultry food safety systems of exporting countries to be equivalent to the US system (GAO, 1998). FDA lacks the authority to require that imported foods be produced under a system equivalent to the one that it administers domestically; instead, FDA relies primarily on sampling at ports-of-entry to determine whether food imports meet domestic requirements (GAO, 1998). Even if FDA's criteria for sampling and testing were systematically risk-based and its resources were adequate to keep up with a growing demand, sample analysis is not capable of detecting many of the most serious risks to consumer health.

In fact, although both agencies have computerized systems to assist in inspection and tracking, there is no way to determine whether the agencies are focusing their attention on the most important health risks. Both agencies target resources to meet the problems of past violations, in which contamination, processing defects, labeling, and quality were at issue.

The General Accounting Office has reported that FDA lacks the necessary controls over detained and suspect shipments (GAO, 1998). Unscrupulous importers are able to circumvent the system, and are seldom punished in proportion to the seriousness of their violations. Similar concerns center on fish and shellfish inspection as over 50 percent of the fish and shellfish consumed in the United Sates is imported (GAO, 1998). It has been reported that shellfish alone caused 21 percent of all reported foodborne illnesses from 1978 to 1992 (CDC, personal communication to committee, June 1998).

In an effort to address the challenges of ensuring the safety of imported foods, the President has proposed a variety of measures including hiring additional FDA inspectors to examine the safety of US fruits and vegetables, both domestic and imported. In addition, legislation is being proposed to allow FDA to halt imports of fruits, vegetables, and other food products that do not meet US food safety requirements or that do not provide the same level of protection as is required for US products. Recognizing that sample analysis does not provide a means for detecting many of the most serious risks to consumer health, and without firm knowledge of most significant risks, it is impossible to know whether the proposed actions will adequately address imported food hazards.

SUMMARY FINDINGS: Where the US Food Safety System Falls Short

- Inconsistent, uneven and at times archaic food statutes that inhibit use of science-based decision-making in activities related to food safety, including imported foods;
- a lack of adequate integration among the 12 primary federal agencies that are involved in implementing the 35 primary statutes that regulate food safety;
- inadequate integration of federal programs and activities with state and local activities;
- absence of focused leadership: no single federal entity is both responsible for the government's efforts and given the authority to implement policy and designate resources toward food safety activities;
- lack of similar missions with regard to food safety of the various agencies reviewed;
- inadequate emphasis on surveillance necessary to provide timely information on current and potential foodborne hazards;
- resources currently identified for research and surveillance are inadequate to support a science-based system;
- limited consumer knowledge, which does not appear to have much impact on food-handling behavior; and
- lack of nationwide adherence to appropriate minimum standards.

6

Conclusions and Recommendations

Congress commissioned the National Academy of Sciences, through the US Department of Agriculture's (USDA) Agricultural Research Service, to undertake the study that resulted in this report. The charge to the committee was to perform two main tasks: assess the current US food safety system and its effectiveness in addressing the continually changing concerns about food safety; and provide recommendations on scientific and organizational changes needed to ensure an effective food safety system for the present and future generations.

The effectiveness of efforts to ensure the safety of food for US consumers is not solely, perhaps not even primarily, the responsibility of the federal government. An effective food safety system depends on the collective efforts of food producers, processors, transporters, suppliers, preparers, retailers, and handlers; of officials at the local, state, and federal levels; and of consumers who select and prepare food. There are three overriding conclusions that the committee came to as a result of its deliberations:

I. **An effective and efficient food safety system must be based on science.**

II. **To achieve a food safety system based on science, current statutes governing food safety regulation and management must be revised.**

III. **To implement a science-based system, reorganization of federal food safety efforts is required.**

The committee's recommendations focus on two main areas. The first addresses the scientific basis of prudent, cost-effective food safety regulation. The second addresses the legal framework and management structure within which the scientific basis should be developed and deployed. The committee presents these recommendations as an integrated, mutually reinforcing package. Specifically, the committee believes that the development and, critically, the use of a scientifically supportable foundation for regulation is not likely to be achieved within the current scattered organization of federal food safety programs, where responsibility is dispersed, budgets are separate, a unified mission is lacking, and no single official has formal or public overall responsibility and authority for performance.

More study is needed to determine the best organizational plan for a centrally unified framework for managing the federal system. The committee's recommendations do not assume that the only way to improve food safety is to create a single responsible agency. The committee also recognizes that designing the details of a centrally managed federal system will generate controversy and will in any case take time. Moreover, it should be emphasized that many of the specific elements of its recommendations can and should be implemented without waiting for the creation of a centrally managed federal system.

The committee emphasizes the urgency of reform,[1] both scientific and organizational. Threats to the safety of food consumed by Americans are ubiquitous and, whether or not the threats are growing, they are certainly changing. Diverse observers of the food safety system, including entities attached to both Congress and the White House, have been calling attention to specific gaps and deficiencies for more than a decade (see Appendix B for a description of previous proposals related to changes in organizational structure). Responsive legislative and administrative actions along the lines of those recommended are long overdue.

SCIENTIFIC RECOMMENDATIONS

Recommendation I:

Base the food safety system on science.

The United States has enjoyed notable successes in improving food safety. An example of these is the joint government-industry development of low-acid

---

[1]During the 1 month period in which the final committee meeting was held (June, 1998), national public health officials in the US reported three major outbreaks involving collectively more than 7,000 reported cases of food-related illness. It is assumed that many more cases of food-related illnesses occurred during this time period as most foodborne illnesses are either unreported or unrecognized as part of an outbreak.

canned food regulations, based on contingency microbiology and food engineering principles, that has almost eliminated botulism resulting from improperly processed commercial food. Similarly, the passage of the 1958 Food Additives Amendment to the Food, Drug, and Cosmetics Act of 1938 was a "technology forcing" event that improved the evaluation of the safety of added and natural substances and reduced the risks associated with the use of food additives. With increasing knowledge, many rational, science-based regulatory philosophies have been adopted, some of which rely on quantitative risk assessment. Adoption of this regulatory philosophy has been uneven and difficult to ensure given the fragmentation of food safety activities, and the differing missions of the various agencies responsible for specific components of food safety. This philosophy must be integrated into all aspects of the food safety system, from federal to state and local.

The greatest strides in ensuring food safety from production to consumption can be made through a scientific risk-based system that ensures that surveillance, regulatory, and research resources are allocated to maximize effectiveness. This will require identification of the greatest public health needs through surveillance and risk analysis. The state of knowledge and technology defines what is achievable through the application of current science. Public resources can have the greatest favorable effect on public health if they are allocated in accordance with the combined analysis of risk assessment and technical feasibility. It is important to recognize that limiting allocation of resources to *only* those areas where high priority hazards exist can create another problem: other hazards with somewhat lower priority but with a much greater probability of reduction or elimination will not be addressed due to limited resources. Thus, both the relative risks and benefits must be considered in allocating resources.

Recommendation IIa:

Congress should change federal statutes so that inspection, enforcement, and research efforts can be based on scientifically supportable assessments of risks to public health.

At a minimum, Congress should legislatively modify the provisions of the Meat Inspection Act and the Poultry Products Inspection Act that are now understood to require physical inspection of each animal carcass and thereby force resources to be allocated in a fashion that is not calibrated to risk. Adequate resources should be made available for the implementation of the Hazard Analysis Critical Control Point (HACCP) system by the USDA and the Food and Drug Administration.

Resource allocations should be subject to revision and adjustment as assessments of risk change. Implementing a food safety system based on risk assessment will require a new level of flexibility in statutory directives to permit responsiveness to advances in science and technology that underlie the food system and food safety efforts.

BOX 6-1.   Changes in Federal Statutes that Would Foster and Enhance Science-Based Strategies

*   Eliminate continuous inspection system for meat and poultry and replace with a science-based approach which is capable of detecting hazards of concern;
*   mandate a single set of science-based inspection regulations for all foods; and
*   mandate that all imported foods come from only countries with food safety standards deemed equivalent to US standards.

Recommendation IIb:

Congress and the administration should require development of a comprehensive national food safety plan. Funds appropriated for food safety programs (including research and education programs) should be allocated in accordance with science-based assessments of risk and potential benefit.

The National Food Safety Plan should:

*   Include a unified, science-based food safety mission;
*   integrate federal, state, and local food safety activities;
*   allocate funding for food safety in accordance with science-based assessments of risk and potential benefit;
*   provide adequate and identifiable support for research and surveillance to:
    —   monitor changes in risk or potential hazards brought on by changes in the food supply or consumption patterns, and
    —   improve the capability to predict and avoid new hazards;
*   increase monitoring and surveillance efforts to improve knowledge of the incidence, seriousness, and cause-effect relationships of foodborne disease and related hazards;
*   address the additional and distinctive efforts required to ensure the safety of imported foods;
*   recognize and provide support for the burdens imposed on state and local authorities that have primary front-line responsibility for the regulation of food service establishments; and
*   address consumers' behaviors related to safe food-handling practices.

RATIONALE FOR RECOMMENDATIONS RELATED TO
A SCIENCE-BASED SYSTEM

The greatest strides in ensuring food safety from production to consumption can be made through a scientific risk-based system that ensures that surveillance, regulatory, and research resources are allocated to maximize effectiveness. That will require identification of the greatest public health needs and greatest opportunities for improvement through prevention, surveillance and risk analysis. The state of knowledge and technology defines what is achievable through the application of current science. Public resources can have the greatest favorable effect on public health if they are allocated in accordance with the combined analysis of risk assessment and technical feasibility.

Both risks and scientific understanding of risks change, so federal efforts must be carried out within a flexible framework. US regulatory agencies are moving toward science-based HACCP programs. The committee found evidence that current resources might be inadequate both to continue traditional inspection and to implement HACCP systems fully. A glaring defect in the present system is that substantial resources are directed to problems that do not have the greatest human health impact (for example, carcass-by-carcass organoleptic [primarily visual and odor detection] inspection of meat and poultry).

The elimination of continuous inspection for meat and poultry would not necessarily end all ante- or postmortem inspections of carcasses, if HACCP programs were appropriately developed and implemented. Such programs would have to include appropriate methods to identify diseased animals, which might require some level of carcass inspection as identified by hazard analysis.

Current understanding of the magnitude of the problem of foodborne disease and the importance of the relevant hazards is incomplete and in many cases inaccurate. Furthermore, there is a lack of scientific resources and structure to address the gaps and inaccuracies. Effective and adequate monitoring, surveillance, and research to characterize risk are required to improve the allocation of resources and to develop the knowledge and technology needed to manage hazards that pose the greatest risk.

The committee found many instances in which the resource base for research and surveillance was not adequate to achieve the critical goals discussed. There is not an adequately coordinated effort on the scale required to analyze the risks and respond to the challenges presented by the changing nature of American food hazards related to increases in consumption of imported foods and in meals eaten away from home.

It is also important that any national plan directly address the safety of imported food. Not all agencies responsible for monitoring the safety of imported food are authorized to enter into agreements with the governments of exporting countries in order to reciprocally recognize food safety standards or inspection results. Uniform or harmonized food safety standards or practices should be encouraged, and officials allowed to undertake research, monitoring, surveillance, or inspection activities within other countries. This should permit inspection and monitoring efforts to be allocated in accordance with science-based analyses of risk and benefit.

The committee found two major problems with respect to consumer education: in some instances, consumer knowledge is inadequate or erroneous; and even where knowledge is adequate, it often fails to influence behavior. A task force to examine approaches to and resources for consumer education is required.

Role of Risk Analysis

The cornerstone of a science-based system of food safety is the incorporation of the results of risk analysis into all decisions regarding resource allocation, programmatic priorities, and public education activities. Risk assessment integrates data on exposure to harmful agents and dose-response relationships to estimate the risk of developing illness from eating specific foods. The growing acceptance of the principles of risk assessment has also led to its use beyond regulatory standard-setting. It is now possible to use comparisons of risk to inform and set priorities for risk management. Risk-based priorities enable resources to be so allocated as to protect public health and to attack the worst problems and/or those most amenable to change first.

Resources Required for Research

To move from a reactive mode of research based on responses to food safety crises to a preventive mode in which newly emerging hazards are identified, or, if possible, prevented, and potential methods for containment evaluated, the federal agency(ies) responsible for food safety regulation will need authority to direct the allocation of funds for food safety research. Intramural and extramural research priorities should be focused on both short- and long-term hazard prevention and on advancing understanding of foodborne pathogens and other food-related hazards; research results should then be integrated into the standard-setting and regulatory program. Selection of research priorities should be based on identification of the greatest potential areas for foodborne risks and assessment of the likely contributions of research findings to the prevention of illness and the improvement of regulatory performance.

In addition to research targeted at immediate regulatory needs, there should continue to be a federally supported, long-term, strategic research program. It should have both applied and basic components and be targeted at the needs of producers, processors, consumers, and nonregulatory and regulatory scientists.

RECOMMENDATIONS TO IMPLEMENT A SCIENCE-BASED SYSTEM THROUGH ORGANIZATIONAL CHANGES

Recommendation IIIa:

To implement a science-based system, Congress should establish, by statute, a unified and central framework for managing federal food safety programs, one that is headed by a single official and which has the responsibility and control of resources for all federal food safety activities, including outbreak management, standard-setting, inspection, monitoring, surveillance, risk assessment, enforcement, research, and education.

The committee was asked to look at organizational changes that would improve the safety of food in the United States. In the time available for information gathering and deliberation, the committee identified characteristics needed in an organizational structure that would improve food safety in the United States. The committee found that the current fragmented regulatory structure is not well-equipped to meet the current challenges. The committee's key recommendation is that to achieve a structure that can implement a science-based system, one official should be responsible for federal efforts in food safety and have control of the resources allocated to food safety.

This recommendation contemplates a structure that would have an identifiable, high-ranking, presidentially appointed head, who would direct and coordinate federal activities and speak to the nation, giving federal food safety efforts a single voice. The structure created, and the person heading it, should have control over the resources Congress allocates to the food safety effort; the structure should also have a firm foundation in statute and thus not be easily subject to changes in political agendas. It is also important that the person heading the structure should be accountable to an official no lower than a cabinet-level secretary, and ultimately, to the President.

Whether or not a single agency emerges, the ultimate structure must provide for not just delegated responsibility, but also for control of resources and authority over food safety activities in the federal government

Recommendation IIIb:

Congress should provide the agency responsible for food safety at the federal level with the tools necessary to integrate and unify the efforts of authorities at the state and local levels to enhance food safety.

This report specifically addresses the federal role in the food safety system, but the roles of state and local government entities are equally critical. For integrated operation of a food safety system, officials at all levels of government must work together in support of common goals of a science-based system. The federal government must be able to ensure nationwide adherence to minimal standards when it is deemed appropriate. The work of the states and localities in support of the federal mission deserves improved formal recognition and appropriate financial support.

BOX 6-2.   Statutory Tools Required to Integrate Local and State Activities Regarding Food Safety into an Effective National System

- Authority to mandate adherence to minimal federal standards for products or processes,
- continued authority to deputize state and local officials to serve as enforcers of federal law,
- funding to support, in whole or in part, activities of state and local officials that are judged necessary or appropriate to enhance the safety of food,
- authority given to the federal official responsible for food safety to direct action by other agencies with assessment and monitoring capabilities, and
- authority to convene working groups, create partnerships, and direct other forms and means of collaboration to achieve integrated protection of the food supply.

RATIONALE FOR ORGANIZATIONAL RECOMMENDATIONS

Centralized and Unified Federal Framework

The committee believes that the creation of a centralized and unified federal framework is critical to improve the food safety system. Many members of the committee are of the view that the most viable means of achieving the goal would be a single, unified agency headed by a single administrator—an agency that would incorporate the several relevant functions now dispersed, and in many instances separately organized, among three departments and a department-level agency. However, in the time frame given the committee, it was not possible to determine whether this is the only sound approach or whether the costs of achieving it would be too high. Nor was it the committee's charge to resolve these issues.

The committee did discuss some possible structures; while it ruled out some, it certainly did not examine all possible configurations and thus the examples provided below are only illustrative of possible overall structures that could be considered. The committee does not believe that the type of centralized focus envisioned can be achieved through the appointment of an individual with formal coordinating responsibility but without legal authority or budgetary control for food safety, a model similar to a White House-based "czar". Nor, in the committee's view, can this goal be achieved through a coordinating committee similar to that currently provided via the National Food Safety Initiative. Experience indicates that any ad hoc administrative adjustments and commitments to coordinate will not suffice to bring about the cultural changes and collaborative efforts needed to create an integrated system.

In evaluating possible structures, the committee realized that past experience with other structures or reorganizations, including the creation of new agencies, such as the Environmental Protection Agency, should inform any final judgment. Further, it is quite possible that other models may now exist in government that can serve as templates for an improved structure. It thus proposes that a sequential, detailed examination of specific organizational changes be a major component of future study, in keeping with the Congressional appropriations language.

**BOX 6-3.   Some Examples of Possible Organizational Structures
to Create a Single Federal Voice for Food Safety**

- A Food Safety Council with representatives from the agencies with a central chair appointed by the President, reporting to Congress and having control of resources,
- designating one current agency as the lead agency and having the head of that agency be the responsible individual,
- a single agency reporting to one current cabinet-level secretary, and
- an independent single agency at cabinet level.

NOTE: These examples are provided for illustrative purposes and many other configurations are possible. It is strongly recommended that future activities be directed toward identifying a feasible structure that meets the criteria outlined.

Integration of Food Safety Efforts

This report specifically addresses the federal role in the food safety system, but the roles of state and local government entities are equally critical. For integrated operation of the food safety system, officials at all levels of government must work together in support of common goals. The federal government must be able to ensure nationwide adherence to minimal standards. The work of the states and localities in support of the federal mission deserves better formal recognition and appropriate financial support.

Similarly, the increased demand of US consumers for year-round availability of fruits and vegetables and the internationalization of the food supply generally have created an increased need for regulatory inspection and control of imported foods. Rationalization of an expanded system of import controls should be based on risk analysis and rely on greatly increased cooperation with US trading partners.

The food industry, from production to delivery, must be included in the planning and implementation of comprehensive food safety efforts. Consumers also have the crucial responsibility of knowing and practicing safe food-handling procedures to protect themselves and their families. Government officials should develop and support partnerships and joint activities with the food industry and with consumers in pursuit of the goal of combating foodborne illness and related hazards.

References

Archer DL, Kvenberg JE. 1985. Incidence and cost of foodborne diarrheal disease in the United States. *J Food Prot* 48(10):887–894.

Bock SA. 1992. The incidence of severe adverse reactions to food in Colorado. *J Allergy Clin Immunol* 90(4 Pt 1):683–685.

Buzby JC, Roberts T. 1997. Guillain–barre syndrome increases foodborne disease costs. *Food Rev* 20(3):36–42.

CAST(Council for Agricultural Science and Technology). 1994. *Foodborne pathogens: risks and consequences.* Council for Agricultural Science and Technology, Ames, IA.

CFIA(Canadian Food Inspection Agency). 1997. *Corporate business plan, 1997–2000.*

CFIA. 1998. *1998–99 Report on plans and priorities.*

Consumers Union. 1998. Chicken: What you don't know can hurt you. *Consumer Reports.* March 1998. pp. 12–18.

Dale K, Wildavsky A. 1991. Individual differences in risk perception and risk–taking preferences.(pp. 15–24) In *The Analysis, Communication and Perception of Risk.* BJ Garrick and WC Gekler, eds. Plenum Press, New York, NY.

DeWaal CS, Dahl E. 1997. Adoption of the 1995 food code: A survey of 45 state and local health departments. *J Assoc Food Drug Officials.* 61(4):15–29.

DHHS(Department of Health and Human Services). 1995. *Food Code.* Public Health Service, Food and Drug Administration. Department of Commerce, Springfield, VA.

DHHS. 1997a. *Food Code.* Public Health Service, Food and Drug Administration. US Department of Commerce, Springfield, VA.

DHHS. 1997b. FDA approves irradiation of meat and pathogen control. *HHS News,* Dec 2, 1997. US Department of Health and Human Services, Washington, DC.

DHHS. 1998. National computer network in place to combat foodborne illness. *HHS News*, May 22, 1998. US Department of Health and Human Services, Washington, DC.

Douglas M, Wildavsky A. 1982. *Risk and Culture*. University of California Press, Berkeley, CA.

Douglas M. 1985. *Risk Acceptability According to the Social Sciences. Social Research Perspectives*. Russell Sage Foundation, New York, NY.

FAO/WHO(Food and Agriculture Organization of the United Nations/World Health Organization). 1997. Codex Alimentarius Commission: Procedural Manual, *Tenth Edition*. Joint FAO/WHO Food Standards Programme, FAO, Rome.

FDA(Food and Drug Administration). 1995. Procedures for the safe and sanitary processing and importing of fish and fishery products, final rule. Food and Drug Administration, Department of Health and Human Services. *Fed Reg* 60(242):65095–65202.

Federal Coordinating Council for Science, Engineering, and Technology. 1993. *An Overview of Food Safety Research. A report by the Committee on Food, Agricultural, and Forestry Research*. Washington, DC.

Fitchen J. 1987. Cultural aspects of environmental problems: individualism and chemical contamination of groundwater. *Sci Tech Hum Values*. 12(2):1–12.

FMI(Food Marketing Institute). 1997a. *Mealtime trends: the state of dinnertime solutions, vol. 1*. Food Marketing Institute, Washington, DC.

FMI. 1997b. *Food marketing industry speaks and detailed tabulations*. Food Marketing Institute, Washington, DC.

FMI. 1998a. *Trends in the United States: Consumer attitudes and the supermarket, 1998*. Food Marketing Institute, Washington, DC.

FMI. 1998b. *A study of consumer trends toward irradiation*. Food Marketing Institute, Washington, DC.

Francer JK, Jung CH, Pak SS. 1998. *Food safety: Enhancing a fragmented regulatory system*. John F. Kennedy School of Government, Harvard University, Cambridge, MA.

FSIS(Food Safety and Inspection Service). 1996a. *Food Standards and Labeling Policy Book*. US Department of Agriculture, Washington, DC.

FSIS. 1996b. Pathogen reduction; Hazard analysis and critical control point systems, final rule. United States Department of Agriculture. *Fed Reg* 61(144):38806–38989.

FSIS. 1997. *Hazard analysis and critical control point(HACCP) update. June 17, 1997*. US Department of Agriculture, Washington, DC.

FSIS. 1998. *HACCP implementation. A science–based strategy for protecting the public health*. U.S. Department of Agriculture, Washington, DC.

GAO(U.S. General Accounting Office). 1992. Food safety and quality. Uniform, risk–based inspection system needed to ensure safe food supply. Report to the Chairman, Subcommittee on Oversight and Investigations, Committee on Energy and Commerce, US House of Representatives. Resources, Community, and Economic Division, *Report 92–152*. Washington, DC.

GAO. 1994a. Food safety: Risk–based inspections and microbial monitoring needed for meat and poultry. Resources, Community and Economic Division, *Report 94–110*. Washington, DC.

GAO. 1994b. Food Safety: Changes needed to minimize unsafe chemicals in food. *Report 94–192*. Washington, DC.

GAO. 1997. Food Safety: Fundamental changes needed to improve food safety. *Report 97–249*. Washington, DC.

GAO. 1998. Food safety: Federal efforts to ensure the safety of imported foods are inconsistent and unreliable. Resources, Community and Economic Division, *Report 98–103*. Washington, DC.

Groth E. 1991. Communicating with consumers about food safety and risk issues. *Food Tech* 45(5):248–253.

Guzelian PS, Henry CJ, Olin SS(eds). 1992. *Similarities and differences in adults and children: Implications for safety assessment*. ILSI Press, Washington, DC.

Hartman and New Hope. 1998. *U.S. consumer use of vitamins, minerals, and herbal supplements: VMHS phase one*. Hartman & New Hope, Bellevue, WA.

Hefle SL, Nordlee JA, Taylor SL. 1996. Allergenic Foods. *Crit Rev Food Sci Nutr* 36–Suppl:S69–89.

Hennessy TW, Hedberg CW, Slutsker L, White KE, Besser–Wiek JM, Moen ME, Feldman J, Coleman WW, Edmonson LM, MacDonald KL, Osterholm MT, The Investigation Team. 1996. A national outbreak of *Salmonella enteritidis* infections from ice cream. *N Engl J Med* 334:1281–6.

IFIC(International Food Information Council Foundation). 1998. *Food for thought II: Reporting of diet, nutrition and food safety*. Washington, DC.

ILSI(International Life Sciences Institute). 1996. *Critical Reviews in Food Science and Nutrition, Special Supplement – Allergenicity of Foods Produced by Genetic Modifications*, F. Clydesdale(ed.), vol. 36:S1–186.

IFT. 1998. Guiding principles for optimum food safety oversight and regulation in the United States. *Food Tech* 52(5):30, 50–52.

IOM(Institute of Medicine). 1997. *Dietary reference intakes: Calcium, phosphorus, magnesium, vitamin D, and fluoride*. National Academy Press, Washington, DC.

Kuhn TS. 1970(1962). *The structure of scientific revolutions*, second edition, enlarged. The University of Chicago Press, Chicago, IL.

Lowrance WW. 1976. *Of acceptable risk*. W. Kaufmann, Inc. Los Altos, CA.

Maciorowski KG, Nisbet DJ, Ha SD, Corrier DE Jr, Ricke SC. 1997. Fermentation and growth response of a primary poultry isolate of *Salmonella typhimurium* grown under strict anaerobic conditions in continuous culture and amino acid–limited batch culture. *Adv Exp Med Biol* 412:201–208.

MAFF(Ministry of Agriculture, Fisheries, and Food). 1998. *The food standards agency: A force for change*. London, England.

Miller SA. 1997. Developing a new food wholesomeness science to ensure food safety. *Food Tech* 51(12):62–65.

Morris GV, and Potter M. 1997. Emergence of new pathogens as a function of changes in host susceptibility. *Emerg Infect Dis* 3(4):435–441.

NAS(National Academy of Sciences). 1987. *Poultry inspection: The basis for a risk assessment approach*. National Academy Press, Washington, DC.

NAS. 1990. *Cattle inspection*. National Academy Press, Washington, DC.

NAS. 1993. *Emerging infections: Microbial threats to health in the US*. National Academy Press, Washington, DC.

NASS(National Agricultural Statistics Service). 1995. *Hogs and Pigs*. Agricultural Statistics Board, U.S. Department of Agriculture, Washington, DC.

New Product News. 1998. New product update. January, 1998.

NRC(National Research Council). 1985. *Meat and poultry inspection. The scientific basis of the nation's program.* National Academy Press, Washington, DC.

NRC. 1989. *Improving risk communication.* National Academy Press, Washington, DC.

NRC. 1993. *Pesticides in the diets of infants and children.* National Academy Press, Washington, DC.

NRC. 1994. *Investing in the national research initiative: An update of the competitive grants program in the U.S. Department of Agriculture.* National Academy Press, Washington, DC.

Office of the President. 1998. Press release: *The President announces joint institute for food safety research and labeling of fresh juices. July 4, 1998.* The White House, Washington, DC.

Olson DG. 1998. The irradiation of food. *Food Tech* 52(1):56–62.

OMB(U.S. Office of Management and Budget). 1998. *Budget of the United States, Fiscal Year 1999.*

Osterholm MT, Hedberg CW, Moore KA. In press. Foodborne diseases: Are they really emerging infections? *Emerg Infect Dis.*

Panter EK, Robens JF(eds). 1997. *1997 Progress report on food safety research conducted by ARS.* Agricultural Research Service, United States Department of Agriculture, Washington, DC.

Partnership for Food Safety Education. 1997a. *Backgrounder. Taking the pulse of the general public: Major knowledge gap about foodborne illness prevention.* October 1997.

Partnership for Food Safety Education. 1997b. News Release: *New safe food handling campaign urges Americans to "Fight BAC!"* October 24, 1997.

Putnam JJ, and Allshouse JE. 1997. Food consumption, prices and expenditures, 1970–1995. Food and Consumer Economics Division, Economics Research Service, United States Department of Agriculture, *Statistical Bulletin No. 939*, Washington, DC.

Rawson JM, Vogt DU. 1998. *Food safety agencies and authorities: A primer.* Library of Congress, Congressional Research Service, Washington, DC.

Sandman P. 1987. Risk communication: Facing public outrage. *EPA J* 13(9):21.

Scherer CW. 1991. Strategies for communicating risks to the public. *Food Tech* 45(10):110–116.

Slovic P. 1986. Informing and educating the public about risk. *Risk Anal* 6(4):403–415.

Slovic P. 1987. Perception of risk. *Science* 236(4799):280–285.

Slovic P, Fischhoff B, Lichtenstein S. 1979. Rating the risks. *Environment* 21(3):14–20, 36–39.

Sobal J, Kahn LK, Bisogni CA. In press. A conceptual model of the food and nutrition system. *Soc Sci Med.*

United States Census Bureau. 1997. Data base news in aging. *Federal Interagency Forum on Aging–Related Statistics.* United States Census Bureau, Washington, DC.

USDA(United States Department of Agriculture). 1939. *Food and life.* United States Department of Agriculture, Washington, DC.

Wolf I. 1992. Critical issues in food safety, 1991–2000. *Food Tech* 46(1):64–70.

A

Glossary and Organizational Framework

for

the Current Food Safety System

A.1

Glossary of Acronyms and Abbreviations

AMS—Agricultural Marketing Service

APHIS—Animal and Plant Health Inspection Service

ARS—Agricultural Research Service

BATF—Bureau of Alcohol, Tobacco, and Firearms

CDC—Centers for Disease Control and Prevention

CFSAN—Center for Food Safety and Applied Nutrition

CSREES—Cooperative State Research, Education, and Extension Service

CUSTOMS—US Customs Service

CVM—Center for Veterinary Medicine

DHHS—US Department of Health and Human Services

DOC—US Department of Commerce

DOD—US Department of Defence

EPA—US Environmental Protection Agency

ERS—Economic Research Service

FDA—Food and Drug Administration

FS—Under Secretary for Food Safety

FSIS—Food Safety and Inspection Service

FTC—Federal Trade Commission

GIPSA—Grain Inspection, Packers and Stockyards Administration

MRP—Under Secretary for Marketing and Regulatory Programs

NASS—National Agricultural Statistics Service

NCTR—National Center for Toxicological Research

NIH—National Institutes of Health

NMFS—National Marine Fisheries Service

NOAA—National Oceanic and Atmospheric Administration

OECA—Office of Enforcement and Compliance Assistance

OPP—Office of Pesticide Programs

OPPTS—Office of Prevention, Pesticides, and Toxic Substances

ORA—Office of Regulatory Affairs

ORACBA—Office of Risk Assessment and Cost-Benefit Analysis

ORD—Office of Research and Development

REE—Under Secretary for Research, Education and Economics

TREASURY—US Department of Treasury

USDA—US Department of Agriculture

A.2

Major Components of the Current Food Safety System

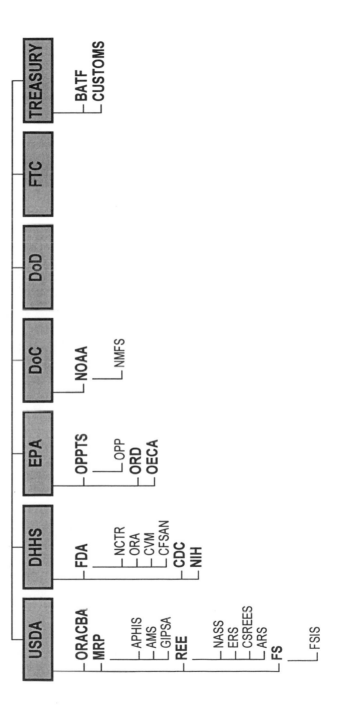

A.3

Federal Food Safety Responsibilities for Selected Food Products and Food Contaminants

Food Safety Activities	Selected Food Products							Food Contaminants	
	Fruits & Vegetables	Dairy Products	Eggs & Egg Products	Meat & Poultry	Seafood	Grain, Rice, & Related Commodities	Imported Foods	Animal Drugs & Feeds	Pesticide Residues
Monitoring/ Surveillance	CDC[a]; CFSAN/ FDA	CDC[a]; CFSAN & CVM/FDA	CDC[a]; CFSAN/ FDA; AMS[b]/ USDA	CDC[a]; CFSAN/ FDA;USDA: FSIS, ERS[c]	CDC[a]; CFSAN/ FDA;NMFS/ NOAA[d]	CDC[a]; CFSAN/ FDA	CDC[a]; CFSAN & ORA/FDA[e]; FSIS/USDA[f]	CDC[a]; CVM/FDA; FSIS/USDA; APHIS	CDC[a]; FSIS/USDA; CFSAN/FDA
Risk Assessment[g]	CFSAN/ FDA; ARS[h]/ USDA	CFSAN; CVM/FDA; ARS[h]/USDA	ARS[h] & FSIS/ USDA; ORACBA; CFSAN/ FDA	USDA: ARS[h], CSREES, FSIS, ERS, ORACBA; CFSAN/FDA	CFSAN/ FDA[i]; NMFS/ NOAA; ARS[h]/USDA	ARS[h]/USDA; CFSAN/ FDA	Same as domestic food products	CVM/FDA; ARS[h]/ USDA; APHIS	OPPTS/EPA[j]; USDA[k]: AMS, ARS[h], ERS, NASS
Research[l]	CFSAN; NCTR/ FDA, USDA: ARS, CSREES[m]	CFSAN; CVM/FDA, CSREES[m] & ARS/USDA	CFSAN/ FDA, ARS/ USDA CSREES[m]	USDA: ARS, CSREES[m]	CVM & CFSAN/ FDA;NMFS/ NOAA; CSREES[m] & ARS/USDA	ARS, CSREES[m]/ USDA; CFSAN/ FDA	Same as domestic food products[n]	CFSAN & CVM/FDA; ARS & CSREES[m] /USDA	ORD/EPA[j]; CSREES[m] & ARS/USDA; CFSAN/FDA

Inspections/ Enforcement	CFSAN & ORA/FDA	CFSAN, ORA, & CVM/FDA	FSIS[o]/ USDA; FDA: CVM, CFSAN, & ORA	FSIS/USDA; CFSAN[p] & CVM/FDA	ORA & CFSAN/ FDA; NMFS/ NOAA[q]	GIPSA[r]/ USDA; ORA & CFSAN/FDA	FSIS[s]/ USDA; CFSAN & ORA/FDA[s]	ORA & CVM/FDA; FSIS[t]/ USDA; APHIS[u]	USDA[v]: FSIS, AMS;FDA[v]: CFSAN, CVM, & ORA; OECA/EPA
Education	CFSAN/ FDA; CSREES[m], ARS[w]/ USDA	CFSAN/ FDA; CSREES[m], ARS[w]/USDA	CFSAN FDA; FSIS & CSREES[m], ARS[w]/ USDA	USDA: FSIS, CSREES[m], ARS[w], ERS[x], ORACBA[x]; CFSAN/FDA	CFSAN/ FDA; CSREES[m], ARS[w]/ USDA; NMFS/ NOAA[y]	CSREES[m], ARS[w]/ USDA; CFSAN/FDA	CSREES[m], ARS[w]/ USDA; CFSAN/ FDA	CSREES[m], ARS[w]/USDA; CVM/FDA	CFSAN/FDA; FSIS & CSREES[m] ARS[w]/USDA

SOURCES: Appendix C; Emilie Cole, NMFS, personal communication, July 1998; EPA, personal communication, July 1998; EPA, personal communication to committee, May 1998; FDA, personal communication to committee, May 1998; Francer et al., 1998; GAO, 1998; Karen Hulabek, FDA, personal communication, July 1998; Edward Knipling, USDA, personal communication, July 1998; July Nelson, EPA, personal communication, July 1998; Morris Potter, CDC, personal communication to committee, May 1998

[a] CDC assists state and Federal agencies in investigating outbreaks of foodborne illness, monitors information on foodborne illness, and conducts research and education related to these illnesses.

[b] AMS operates the shell egg surveillance program to visually detect physical damage or conditions which, in turn, might subject eggs to hazardous organisms.

[c] ERS utilizes data collected by FoodNet to analyze the costs associated with foodborne illness and the benefits of improving food safety.

[d] Most product monitoring is not to determine individual lot compliance, but rather to provide scientific oversight and system surveillance of the DOC inspection program.

[e] FDA uses several sources of information to monitor imported food shipments: FDA's Import Alert Retrieval System database contains a list of products that FDA automatically detains because the exporter or the specific food products have shown a history of violations in previous shipments. FDA's Low-Acid Canned Food database contains information on foreign processors of low-acid and acidified canned foods registered with FDA. FDA's Operational and Administrative System for Import Support (OASIS) contains information on products that are not automatically released into domestic commerce.

[f] FSIS maintains a centralized computer system, Automated Import Information System (AIIS), which contains information on the exporting country, plant, and eligibility of product.

[g] Risk assessment responsibilities include implementation of science-based tools for minimizing the occurrence of foodborne hazards such as setting standards for pesticide residues. In FY 1997, FDA, USDA, and EPA established an interagency risk assessment consortium at the Joint Institute of Food Safety and Applied Nutrition at the University of Maryland.

[h] ARS provides data for all food product and contaminant areas to support risk assessment by FSIS, ERS, ORACBA, FDA, and EPA.

[i] FDA has the authority to set tolerances in seafood and all other foods except meat and poultry for natural and synthetic contaminants, except for pesticides, which are set by EPA.

[j] The public responsibilities of EPA's pesticide program include other activities unrelated to food safety such as: protection of workers, communities from pesticide drift, families from residues from house and garden applications and children from unintentional ingestion of pesticides.

k AMS, ARS, ERS, and NASS are involved in data collection to support the pesticide risk assessment process. AMS manages the Pesticide Data Program (data collection) to support the pesticide risk assessment activity by other agencies.

l NIH also does research on food safety problems, however, it is not listed as food safety research. NIH research is targeted as human health issues regardless of the mechanism.

m USDA formula funds provided by CSREES to the Land Grant Universities broadly support research and education activities across all food product areas.

n For imported foods, ARS develops methodology to detect contaminants and residues as necessary in support of agencies with surveillance and inspection responsibilities.

o FSIS is responsible for inspecting all egg products used by manufacturers, food service, and retail markets. FDA is responsible for inspecting shell eggs, egg substitutes, imitation eggs, and similar products).

p CFSAN has responsibility for inspection/enforcement of game meats.

q NMFS runs a voluntary inspection service.

r GIPSA has responsibility for monitoring the accuracy of aflatoxin testing services.

s The FSIS in USDA is responsible for imported meat, poultry, and some egg products. The FDA is responsible for all other imported foods.

t FSIS is responsible for the inspection of meat and poultry products in Federally-inspected establishments and reports violative residues of drugs in meat and poultry to FDA for regulatory follow-up. FSIS has authority to condemn carcasses having violative drug residues. FDA conducts follow-up inspections of producers or others involved in the production or marketing of food animals or poultry which have tissue residue violations. The goal of CVM's Tissue Residue Program is to eliminate violative drug residues in edible tissue of food animals. Because of resource constraints, FDA cannot investigate all of the initial tissue residue violations reported by FSIS.

u APHIS carries out U.S. border quarantine activities to detect and eliminate animal health problems and exotic organisms that might harm U.S. agriculture, many of which also pose potential food safety threats.

v USDA's FSIS is responsible for monitoring pesticide residues in meat, poultry, and certain egg products. USDA's AMS, through contracts, has carried out a residue testing program directed primarily at raw agricultural products. AMS also manages the Pesticide Recordkeeping Program (data collection) for Federally restricted-use pesticides. FSIS and AMS report their pesticide residue data independently. FDA's CFSAN is responsible for enforcing pesticide tolerances in all imported foods and domestically produced foods shipped in interstate commerce. FDA's CVM directs the portion of the Agency's pesticide monitoring program concerned with domestic and imported animal feeds for pesticide residues. This is via CVM's Feed Contaminants Compliance Program.

w ARS provides information resources via the National Agricultural Library to the public, industry, universities, and other government agencies. ARS technical employees participate in educational and technology transfer workshops attended by other scientists from industry, university, and government.

x ERS and the ORACBA provide technical assistance to identify education needs and to analyze the effectiveness of food safety education programs.

y Seafood HACCP training

A.4

Federal Food Safety Responsibilities by Agency

Food Safety Activities	MRP/USDA	REE/USDA	ORACBA/USDA	FSIS/USDA	FDA/HHS	CDC/HHS	NIH/HHS	EPA	NMFS/NOAA/DOC
Monitoring/ Surveillance	**APHIS AMS:** egg and egg products			FoodNet system [a] Conducts pesticide residue, drug residue, pathogen, & BSE monitoring	**CFSAN:** FoodNet system [a]; **CVM:** NASMP [b]	Lab surveillance; passive surveillance of outbreaks[c]; FoodNet system [a]			Seafood
Risk Assessment	**APHIS AMS:** pesticides [d]	**ARS** [e] **CSREES:** meat & poultry **ERS:** meat, poultry, pesticides [d] **NASS:** pesticides [d]	Eggs, meat, & poultry	meat & poultry; eggs & egg products	CFSAN; **CVM:** dairy products; animal drugs & feeds			**OPPTS:** pesticide residues in food; pesticide registration	Seafood[f]

Continued

[a] FoodNet-Foodborne Diseases Active Surveillance Network, jointly developed by FSIS, CDC, & FDA to collect more precise information on the incidence of foodborne disease.

[b] NASMP-National Antimicrobial Susceptibility Monitoring Program, a collaborative effort among FDA, CDC, & USDA.

[c] CDC assists state & Federal agencies in investigating outbreaks of foodborne illness, monitors information on foodborne illness, & conducts research & education related to these illnesses.

[d] AMS, ERS and NASS are involved in data collection to support the pesticide risk assessment process.

[e] ARS provides data for all food product areas to support risk assessment by FSIS, ERS, ORACBA, FDA, & EPA

[f] Most product monitoring is not to determine individual lot compliance, but rather to provide scientific oversight & system surveillance of the DOC inspection program.

Federal Food Safety Responsibilities by Agency *Continued*

Research	ARS; CSREES[g]	CFSAN:		ORD:
		all food products & contaminants except meat & poultry **CVM:** animal drugs & feeds, dairy products, seafood **NCTR:** fruits & vegetables	epidemiology studies: case-control conducts research on foodborne disease processes and intervention strategies[h]	provide science support for pesticide public health issues seafood
Inspections/ Enforcement	**GIPSA:** grain, rice, & related commodities[i] **APHIS**[j] **AMS:** Pesticide Record-keeping Program[k]	**ORA/CFSAN:** In-plant inspection of all domestic & imported foods (except meat & poultry products)[m] for sale or distribution in interstate commerce; pesticide residues in/on food **CVM:** dairy products; egg & egg products; meat & poultry; animal drugs & feeds; pesticide residues	Inspection of meat, poultry, & egg products[l] for sale or distribution in interstate commerce; reviews foreign plants exporting these products	**OECA:** Voluntary enforcement of seafood pesticide regulations including misuse of pesticides. seafood inspection

Continued

g USDA formula funds provided by CSREES to the L & Grant Universities broadly support research & education activities across all food product areas.

h NIH does research on food safety problems; however, it is not listed as food safety research. NIH research is targeted at human health issues regardless of the mechanism.

i GIPSA has responsibility for monitoring the accuracy of aflatoxin testing services.

j APHIS carries out U.S. border quarantine activities to detect & eliminate animal health problems & exotic organisms that might harm U.S. agriculture, many of which also pose potential food safety threats.

k AMS manages the Pesticide Recordkeeping Program for Federally restricted-use pesticides.

l FSIS is responsible for inspecting all egg products used by manufacturers, food service, & retail markets. FDA is responsible for inspecting shell eggs substitutes, imitation eggs, & similar products.

m CFSAN has responsibility for inspection/enforcement of game meats.

Federal Food Safety Responsibilities by Agency *Continued*

Education				
ARS[n] CSREES[o], [p] ERS[q]	Provides technical assistance to education programs[q]	Collaborative activities[p]; other services: *Meat & Poultry Hotline;* electronic communications[o]	CFSAN: collaborative education activities[p], food labeling, training and technical assistance documents; all food products and contaminants except animal drugs & feeds CVM: animal drugs & feeds	Seafood HACCP training, scientific training/ laboratory training

[n] ARS provides information resources via the National Agricultural Library to the public, industry, universities, & other government agencies. ARS technical employees participate in educational & technology transfer workshops attended by other scientists from industry, university, & government.

[o] FSIS & ARS food safety education activities are conducted by USDA employees, while CSREES supports food safety education activities undertaken by eligible institutions in the land-grant system.

[p] Collaborative educational activities include: Food Safety Education Partnership (which launched "Fight Bac" campaign), a joint effort among USDA, HHS, EPA, the Dept of Education & the private sector; (2) The Food Safety Training & Education Alliance, recently established by FDA, USDA, private sector stakeholders, & consumer advocacy groups.

[q] ERS & the ORACBA provide technical assistance to identify education needs & to analyze the effectiveness of food safety education programs.

B

Food Safety: Recommendations for Changes in the Organization of Federal Food Safety Responsibilities, 1949–1997

April 21, 1998

Donna U. Vogt
Analyst in Social Sciences
Science, Technology, and Medicine Division
Congressional Research Service
The Library of Congress

NOTE: Formatted from a file version received from Donna U. Vogt.

115

ABSTRACT

This report describes recommendations to change the structure of federal food safety responsibilities and gives the reader background information on the debate over the last five decades over which structure would best improve the system for ensuring "safe" food for U.S. consumers. The report lists all the major efforts that were made from 1949 through 1997 by groups inside and outside the federal government. The sets of recommendations are placed chronologically under one of four categories, depending on which organizational structure the group thought would improve food safety. The categories of organization are as follows: an independent single food safety agency, the U.S. Department of Agriculture, or the Food and Drug Administration, or with the Consumer Product Safety Commission. This product will be updated periodically. See also CRS Issue Brief 98009, Food Safety Issues in the 105th Congress.

Food Safety: Recommendations for Changes in the Organization of Federal Food Safety Responsibilities, 1949–1997

SUMMARY

This report summarizes twenty-one sets of recommendations, made in the last five decades, for changing the organization of federal food safety responsibilities. Since 1906, food safety responsibilities and inspections have been split by product under different laws. Congress passed the Pure Food Act and the Meat Inspection Act on June 30, 1906. Both Acts placed the responsibility for food safety in the U.S. Department of Agriculture (USDA), Division of Chemistry (later Bureau). That Bureau later became the Food and Drug Administration. Over time, USDA kept responsibility for meat safety, while most other foods came to be regulated by the Food and Drug Administration (FDA) of the Public Health Service in the Department of Health and Human Services (DHHS).

Recommendations for changing the federal food safety system can be fit into one of four categories. The recommendations proposed that 1) a single, independent institution be given responsibility for all food safety; 2) responsibility for all food products should be returned to USDA; 3) responsibility for all food products should be given to FDA; or 4) responsibility for all food products should be given to the Consumer Product Safety Commission (CPSC).

Most of the recommendations had both supporters and critics. Supporters of the first recommendation claim that the agency could promulgate consistent risk-based regulations and inspections for all types of foods, whether meats or canned foods, and increase the confidence of consumers in the U.S. food supply. Critics claim that a single, independent food safety agency would have large start-up costs in an era of tight budgets and would not be able to take advantage of the long-term experience and regulatory organization developed for different foods by USDA and FDA.

Supporters of the second recommendation claim that USDA could utilize its nationwide network for new research and enforcement. Critics claim that USDA has little institutional culture to support legal regulatory work. They are also concerned that USDA's mission of supporting and promoting agriculture would interfere with its ability to take regulatory action when needed.

Supporters of the third recommendation feel that FDA could use its long-term expertise in combining law and science to regulate consumer products. Critics argue that FDA is not organized to regulate all foods, would have to completely change its orientation, and could be overwhelmed by the process.

Supporters of the fourth recommendation claim that under the CPSC, the fragmented federal authority for food safety could be modernized and focused on protecting U.S. consumers by strengthening the links to federal and state public health departments. Critics are concerned that food is unlike other products that the CPSC has regulated and may not receive the attention it deserves.

Contents

Introduction 121
    Background 121
    Current Federal Food Safety Responsibilities 127
    Overlapping Responsibilities 129
    Recommendations for Changes in the Federal Organization of
        Food Safety Responsibilities 130

Food Safety Under a Single, Independent Agency 132
    White House Conference on Food, 1969 132
    GAO Food Inspection Report, 1970 133
    Hearings on S. 3419, Consumer Safety Act of 1972 134
    Ralph Nader Report, Sowing the Wind, 1972 136
    GAO's Risk Based Inspection Report, 1992 136
    The Durenberger Food Safety Bill, 1993 137
    The Torricelli/Bradley Food Safety Bill, 1994 138
    The Fazio-Durbin Food Safety Administration Bill, 1997 139

Food Safety Under the U.S. Department of Agriculture 140
    The Hoover Commission Report, May 20, 1949 140
    Acts Restructuring Meat and Poultry Products Inspection: Wholesome
        Meat Act of 1967 and the Poultry Products Act of 1968 141

Food Safety Under the Food and Drug Administration 143
    HEW Reorganization Directive of March, 1968 143
    The Malek Report, December 10, 1969 144
    Senate Governmental Affairs Report on Federal Regulation, 1977 145
    President Carter's 1978 Government Reorganization Project or
        White House Study (never released) 146
    Lester Crawford, 1980 147
    Dr. Sanford Miller, 1989 147
    The Edwards FDA Advisory Committee, May 1991 148
    National Performance Review, September 1993 149
    Carol Tucker Foreman, Safe Food Coalition, October 6, 1993 150
    Hearings in Support of the Vice President's National Performance
        Review Recommendations for Reinventing the Food Safety
        System, 1993–1994 152

Food Safety Under the Consumer Product Safety Commission 153
    The Metzenbaum Bill, 1993 153

List of Tables

Table 1. Institutional Chronology of Food Safety Responsibilities,
            1862-1998   126

Table 2. Recommendations for Changes in the Federal Organization of
            Food Safety Responsibilities, 1949–1997   154

Food Safety: Recommendations for Changes in the Organization of Federal Food Safety Responsibilities, 1949–1997[1]

INTRODUCTION

At times, consumers have questioned whether the organization of federal food safety efforts works well enough or whether a different system may better serve consumer needs. Questions often revolve around which standards are used when judging whether food is considered safe, and how the federal government should be organized to respond appropriately to food safety concerns. During the past five decades, those concerns have led the executive branch and Congress to consider recommendations for changes in the organization of federal food safety efforts.

This report summarizes twenty-one sets of recommendations, presented to the President or to Congress between 1949 and 1997 to change the structure of food safety responsibilities. These recommendations were developed by entities inside and outside the federal government. They have included Presidential and other official commissions, Members and committees of Congress, the U.S. General Accounting Office (GAO), and prominent food policy representatives. All recommendations have influenced the debate on restructuring the federal organization of food safety.

Background[2]

The federal government's role in food safety began when safety questions about food were referred to the Division (later Bureau) of Chemistry within a newly created Department of Agriculture (USDA) in the latter half of the nineteenth century. USDA's role began to increase when, at the turn of the century, developments in transportation systems increasingly brought processed food into growing cities. The residents of those cities lost the ability that villagers had possessed of being first-hand judges of the food they ate. U.S. consumers began questioning the safety of what they were buying in stores and expressed concern about the safety of chemical preservatives being used by commercial food processors to extend the life of meats, dairy products, and vegetables, and sometimes to mask their decomposition.

---

[1] CRS Report 93-955, which this report supersedes, was coauthored by Karen L. Alderson, Library Services Division, Congressional Research Service.

[2] Most of the historical material used to prepare this section was provided by Suzanne White Junod, Ph.D., History Office, Food and Drug Administration.

The conditions of some foods led the Bureau of Chemistry to conduct studies of the extent to which adulterated foods had begun to permeate the nation's food supply. While the chief chemist of USDA at that time, Dr. Harvey W. Wiley, estimated that less than 5% of the nation's food was adulterated, he surmised that the overuse of chemical preservatives such as borax, formaldehyde, benzoate of soda, salicylic acid, and copper salts, commonly used as additives in food, could be harmful to health. Those studies convinced Congress to appropriate funds for Dr. Wiley's famous "poison squad." The squad consisted of a group of young men who were given increasing doses of the chemicals to discover their effects on the human metabolism. Many of the young men became ill when they consumed foods containing preservatives in amounts commonly used at that time. The scientific value of the studies remained questionable, but the effect on the public was dramatic when the results were reported. The "poison squad" stories provoked interest in food safety throughout the country. The time was ripe for federal action.

Under pressure from consumer groups and from President Theodore Roosevelt, Congress passed the 1906 Food and Drugs Act on June 30, 1906.[3] That Act set up the regulatory role of the federal government for foods other than meat and poultry by prohibiting from interstate commerce the sale of food and drugs that were adulterated and/or misbranded. Adulteration in the act was defined as

> . . . the intermixture or substitution of substances reducing quality, the abstraction of valuable constituents, the concealment of damage or inferiority, the addition of deleterious ingredients, and the use of spoiled animal or vegetable products.[4]

Misbranding meant placing false or misleading statements on the label. Yet, food safety involved more than adulteration and misbranding. The 1906 Food and Drugs Act also had a provision for enforcement. It required that adulterated foods not only be seized but also destroyed.

In 1905, Upton Sinclair published *The Jungle*, a book about the way meat was mishandled in Chicago's slaughterhouses. It had a major impact on consumers with meat sales falling around the country by nearly a third almost overnight. Congress appointed a commission to examine the charges made in the book. The commission found that while some of the allegations might have been slightly exaggerated, other evidence showed situations actually worse than portrayed by Sinclair. That evidence was used to convince lawmakers to pass the Meat Inspection Act of 1906[5], which set sanitary standards for slaughter of animals and for

---

[3]P.L. 59-384, 34 Stat. 768 (1906).

[4]Lauffer Hayes and Frank Ruff, "The Administration of the Federal Food and Drugs Act," in *Food and Drug Law: Cases and Materials*, ed. Peter Barton Hutt and Richard A. Merrill. 2nd ed. (Westbury, New York: The Foundation Press, Inc., 1991), 9.

[5] P.L. 59-242, 21 U.S.C. §601 et seq.

meat sold in interstate commerce.[6] With the passage of the 1906 Act, USDA began a system of continuous daily inspection in slaughterhouses using organoleptic (sight, smell, touch) means to detect problems. If problems were found, inspectors could instantly condemn carcasses.

With the signing of the 1906 Food and Drugs Act, USDA officials in the Bureau of Chemistry emphasized the development of detection methods to find chemical problems in foods. During the 1920's, conflicts sometimes occurred within the department between officials who were charged with promoting the use of chemicals to produce food and regulators who were concerned about food being adulterated by those chemicals. For example, California apple growers at the time used large quantities of arsenic on apples to fight pests. USDA chemists had set a limit for the maximum amount of arsenic residue that could be left on the fruit. Some of the apples had residues that exceeded that limit. The regulators wanted to declare the apples adulterated; other officials did not.

The conflict in mission began early in the century. The following statement characterizes it:

> The Bureau of Chemistry had originated as a research bureau and law enforcement was a superimposed responsibility. The task of undertaking research designated to improve the methods of utilizing agricultural products was frequently in striking conflict with enforcement of the Pure Food and Drugs law. These conflicts arose, first, because there was a constant tendency to stop a research project so as to permit the scientist to assist in acquiring evidence immediately needed in a lawsuit and second, because the objectives of law enforcement frequently did not coincide with increasing the utilization of a particular agricultural product, but instead might retard its utilization.[7]

In 1927, Dr. Walter Campbell of the Bureau of Chemistry recommended that the Secretary of Agriculture separate the functions of agricultural research and enforcement. At the time, USDA was enforcing several other laws.[8] Campbell

---

[6]Meat had been separated from other food for special legislative treatment in 1890 and 1891. Federal inspection began as a means of reassuring European nations that U.S. meats were safe. Europe had banned imports of U.S. pork on the charge that it had caused epidemics of trichinosis. A newspaper scare arose during the Spanish-American War when U.S. packers were blamed for shipping "embalmed beef" that sickened the troops. Investigation attributed some of the trouble to the rapid growth of bacteria in meat exposed to the hot Cuban sun. James Harvey Young, "The Long Struggle for the 1906 Law," *FDA Consumer*, v. 15, no. 5, June 1981, 16.

[7]Michael Brannon,"Organizing and Reorganizing FDA," in *Seventy-Fifth Anniversary Commemorative Volume of Food and Drug Law,* Food and Drug Law Institute Series, (Washington, D.C., Food Drug Law Institute, 1984), 142.

[8]Laws included the Food and Drugs Act (34 Stat. 768 (1906)), the Insecticide Act (7 U.S.C. §121–134), the Caustic Poison Act (15 U.S.C. §410–411), Naval Stores Act (7

suggested that the Secretary of Agriculture create a Food, Drug, and Insecticide Administration (FDIA) within the Department. Congress supported this suggestion and the 1927 appropriations bill created the FDIA and gave it the responsibility to enforce the 1906 Pure Foods Act.[9] Simultaneously, the Secretary created a soil and chemistry bureau to handle research functions. In 1930, USDA dropped "insecticide" from the agency's title, and its name became the Food and Drug Administration (FDA).

FDA's new enforcement responsibilities continued to grow as did the agency's commitment to consumer protection. In 1930, Congress passed an act setting standards for canned foods, but excluding canned meat and milk products from those standards. As the New Deal began in 1933, pressures mounted to pass a new law that would fill the gaps in the 1906 Pure Food and Drugs Act. A tragedy occurred in 1937 that resulted in strengthening the federal role of premarket review of drugs. At least 73, and perhaps over 90, persons died as a result of taking "Elixir Sulfanilamide." Franklin Roosevelt's son had recovered from a near fatal infection using sulfanilamide, a European wonder drug. Problems developed when the producer began using diethylene glycol as a solvent for sulfanilamide without first determining that the solvent was safe. The disaster prompted passage of the 1938 amendments to the law, requiring manufacturers to prove a drug's safety to FDA before marketing the drug. Consumers began to support the idea that there should be federal premarket approval for both drugs and substances added to foods.

On June 25, 1938, President Roosevelt signed into law the Federal Food, Drug, and Cosmetic Act of 1938[10] (FFDCA) that today remains the basic authorizing legislation for food safety. Even though USDA had primary responsibility for food safety for almost 80 years, the new law defined more clearly USDA's authority to regulate livestock and poultry feeds and drugs used in animal disease control. After the 1938 law was passed, President Roosevelt said,

> "The work of the Food and Drug Administration is unrelated to the basic function of the Department of Agriculture," and he expressed his belief that "the opportunity for the Food and Drug Administration to develop along increasingly constructive lines" lay in the Federal Security Administration.[11]

In 1940, the President moved FDA out of USDA and into the Federal Security Agency (FSA), a separate part of the executive branch. FSA was a new agency; it had been in existence for only one year. At the time, the FSA mission was to protect the public health, and it had under its jurisdiction the Public Health Service,

---

U.S.C. §91 et seq.), Federal Import Milk Act (21 U.S.C. §141 et seq.), Filled Milk Act(21 U.S.C. §61 et seq.), and Tea Importation Act(21 U.S.C. §41 et seq.).

[9] Donald R. Whitnah, ed., *Government Agencies,* (Westport, CT: Greenwood Press, 1983), 251.

[10] 21 U.S.C. §301–392.

[11] Brannon, *Organizing and Reorganizing FDA,* 158.

the Office of Education, the Civilian Conservation Corps, and the Social Security Administration, among other agencies. FDA's responsibilities within the FSA included regulating food quality, sanitation, and consumer protection. Under the new FFDCA, FDA was also given the authority to test the safety of new products and was given research responsibilities. The agency focused on whether a given substance in foods was "poisonous or deleterious" within the meaning of section 406 of the statute. As an operational rule, FDA sought to ban in the diet any substance that proved toxic to laboratory animals at 1% of their diet.

Not everyone agreed with the President's decision about reorganizing FDA. Secretary of Agriculture Henry A. Wallace argued that the meat inspection work of USDA's Bureau of Animal Industry also should be transferred. He claimed,

> This activity might be associated with other health or public welfare work. Meat inspection is of course a technical job and it seems logical to have the technical inspectors attached to the bureau most competent in this field.[12]

However, President Roosevelt was not persuaded; meat and poultry inspection remained within USDA. The USDA meat inspection system had developed on a parallel track within USDA's Bureau of Chemistry for over 50 years. Veterinarians within the Bureau trained inspectors to spot animal diseases. Those inspectors performed continuous inspections of animals before slaughter and examined every carcass for disease and contamination after slaughter. The system positioned the United States to supply meat to the world during World War II.

The war effort was not confined to USDA. Even after FDA was transferred out of USDA, FDA was charged with ensuring the enrichment of breads in 1942 for the soldiers serving in World War II. Several years later (1953), the FSA became the Department of Health, Education, and Welfare (HEW). In 1968, FDA became part of the Public Health Service (PHS) where it added a focus on health and nutrition to its food safety responsibilities.

Since the start of federal regulation, food safety has been the primary responsibility of either of two different cabinet agencies, USDA and Department of Health and Human Services (DHHS). **Table 1** shows which statute and consequently which organization and department has been responsible for carrying out the statutes' mandates for food safety since the federal government became involved.

---

[12]Memo to President Franklin D. Roosevelt from Henry Wallace, 20 April 1939. Found in Senate Committee on Governmental Affairs, "Food Regulation: A Case Study of USDA and FDA," Chapter 4, *Study on Federal Regulation*, 95th Cong., 2nd sess., December 1977, S. Rept. 95-91,140.

Table 1. Institutional Chronology of Food Safety Responsibilities, 1862–1998

Years	Statute/Plan	Name of Organization	Department
1890–1901	Act of March 3, 1891 and Act of March 2, 1895 on exported meats	Division of Chemistry	USDA
1901–1927	1906 Pure Food Act 1906 Appropriations Act	Bureau of Chemistry and Bureau of Animal Industry	USDA
1927–1930	1906 Pure Food Act 1906 Appropriations Act	Food, Drug, and Insecticide Administration	USDA
1930–1940[13]	1938 Federal Food, Drug, and Cosmetic Act (FFDCA)	Food and Drug Administration	USDA
1940–1953	Reorganization Plan No. 4, effective June 3, 1940.	Food and Drug Administration	Federal Security Agency
1953–1970	1954 Miller Pesticide Act and 1958 Food Additives Amendment (Delaney Clause) 1960 Color Additives Amendment (Delaney Clause)	Food and Drug Administration	Department of Health, Education, and Welfare
(1958–1968)	1958 Humane Slaughter Act; 1967 Wholesome Meat Act; 1968 Poultry Products Act	Meat Inspection Branch of Agricultural Research Service	USDA
1970–1979	Reorganization Plan No. 3 of 1970; sect. 346, 346a, 348, and 408 of FFDCA and 135-135k of FIFRA	All pesticide regulation responsibilities were transferred to EPA as were all functions of Environmental Quality Branch, Plant Protection Division of Agricultural Research Service	Environmental Protection Agency (EPA)

[13]The name "Food and Drug Administration" was first used in the Agriculture Appropriation Act of 1931 (46 Stat. 32).

Table 1. *Continued*

Years	Statute/Plan	Name of Organization	Department
(1972)	1972 Meat and Poultry Inspection	Food Safety and Inspection Service	USDA
(1968–1979)	Reorganization Plan of March 1968. Public Health Service Act	Food and Drug Administration Public Health Service	Department of Health, Education, and Welfare
1980–		Food and Drug Administration Public Health Service	Department of Health and Human Services

Source: Peter Barton Hutt and Richard A. Merrill, eds. *Food and Drug Law: Cases and Materials*, 2nd ed., (Westbury, New York: The Foundation Press, Inc., 1991), 4–5.

Current Federal Food Safety Responsibilities

Historically, Congress passed laws in reaction to immediate food safety problems. Those laws assigned food safety responsibilities to several executive departments. Today, the primary federal agencies responsible for regulating the safety of the U.S. food supply are the Food and Drug Administration (FDA) under the Public Health Service of the Department of Health and Human Services (DHHS), and the Food Safety and Inspection Service (FSIS) under the U.S. Department of Agriculture (USDA). FDA and USDA together try to ensure that food products, as sold in the United States, will not adversely affect human health.

FDA is charged with ensuring that foods (except meat, poultry, and certain egg products) are safe, nutritious, sanitary, wholesome, and honestly labeled. The primary statute governing FDA's food safety activities is the Federal Food, Drug, and Cosmetic Act (FFDCA).[14] FDA monitors whether food manufacturers are adhering to their legal responsibility of ensuring that foods are not defective, unsafe, filthy, or produced under unsanitary conditions. USDA is responsible for

---

[14]Other relevant statutes are the Federal Insecticide, Fungicide, and Rodenticide Act (FIFRA), as amended (P.L. 104-61, Stat. 163–172, 1947, 7 U.S.C. §136 et seq.); the Public Health Service Act (Chapter 288, 37 Stat. 309 (1912), 7 U.S.C. §201 et seq.); the Fair Packaging and Labeling Act, as amended (P.L. 89-755, 15 U.S.C. §1451 et seq.); the Federal Meat Inspection Act, as amended (P.L. 90-201, 21 U.S.C. §601 et seq.); the Poultry Products Inspection Act (P.L.85-172, 21 U.S.C. §451 et seq.); Federal Import Milk Act (P.L. 69-625, 21 U.S.C. §141 et seq.); Plant Quarantine Act , as amended (P.L 85-36, 7 U.S.C. §150 et seq.) and the Pesticide Monitoring Improvements Act (P.L.100-418, 21 U.S.C. §1401, et seq.).

monitoring meat, poultry, and commercially processed egg products under the Federal Meat Inspection Act, as amended, the Poultry Products Inspection Act, as amended, and the Egg Products Inspection Act, as amended. FSIS is directly responsible for the daily inspection of all meat and poultry entering U.S. commerce. FSIS also shares responsibility with FDA on combination products such as stews and pizzas. For example, FSIS regulates all products that contain 2% or more of poultry and poultry products and 3% or more of red meat or red meat products. FDA regulates all other foods.

In total, thirteen agencies in the federal government have food safety responsibilities.[15] FDA has three centers conducting and supporting food safety activities: Center for Food Safety and Applied Nutrition (CFSAN), Center for Veterinary Medicine (CVM), and the National Center for Toxicological Research (NCTR). Besides FSIS, the USDA agencies with food safety responsibilities are the Animal and Plant Health Inspection Service (APHIS),which has regulatory programs to protect animals and plants from pests and disease; the Agricultural Research Service (ARS), which conducts a wide range of food safety related research; the Cooperative State Research, Education, and Extension Service (CSREES), which carries out a program of fundamental and applied research in several areas, including food safety and health; and the Economic Research Service (ERS), which provides cost and benefit information on food-borne illnesses. The National Center for Infectious Diseases of the Centers for Disease Control and Prevention (CDC), under DHHS, monitors and investigates food-borne illnesses and diseases and shares that information with the other agencies.

The Environmental Protection Agency (EPA) regulates pesticides and is charged with setting pesticide-residue tolerances for each pesticide-food combination. The Bureau of Alcohol, Tobacco, and Firearms (BATF), of the U.S. Treasury Department, regulates production, distribution, and labeling of alcoholic beverages.[16] The National Marine Fisheries Service (NMFS) of the U.S. Department of Commerce conducts a voluntary fee-for-service seafood inspection program. The Federal Trade Commission (FTC) regulates advertising of food products. The U.S. Customs Service of the Department of the Treasury assists FDA by notifying FDA of incoming shipments of products under FDA jurisdiction. FDA officials examine all paperwork and electronic submissions related to these imports and at times collect samples.

In addition, federal agencies work in close collaboration with state officials. Often, federal agencies such as FDA will train and contract with state enforcement officials to conduct food plant inspections. FDA also developed a model ordinance for milk sanitation and a "Food Code" for retail food store and restaurant sanita-

---

[15]Detailed information on those responsibilities can be found in Congressional Research Service, *Food Safety Agencies and Authorities: A Primer*, by Jean Rawson and Donna U. Vogt, Report No. 98-91 ENR, 5 February 1998, 6.

[16]FDA is responsible for all nonalcoholic beverages, and wine beverages (i.e. fermented fruit juices) containing less than 7% alcohol.

tion to be adopted by state legislatures. FDA also works with groups such as the Association of Food and Drug Officials of the United States and the Association of Official Analytical Chemists.[17] FDA, in conjunction with the states, regulates animal feed ingredients and feeds as part of the American Association of Feed Control Officials.[18]

Overlapping Responsibilities

Critics charge that part of the "food safety problem" is that U.S. food safety laws and regulations are fragmentary and inconsistent and are not comprehensive. Critics also claim that too many agencies are responsible for food safety activities. Foods posing similar health risks may be inspected by different agencies at different frequencies. The roles that these agencies play depend for the most part on their statutory authority and their resources. One former official who served in both USDA and FDA said that the fragmentation and diversity of the agencies' authority undercuts the government's accountability for food safety, and he added:

> FDA has jurisdiction over plants producing cheese pizza, but rarely inspects such plants. USDA has jurisdiction over plants producing pepperoni pizza, and inspects such plants on a daily basis, after having already inspected both the animal from which the pepperoni was made and the processing of the meat into pepperoni.[19]

Other examples abound. USDA daily inspects meat and poultry for contamination of various pathogens, including *Listeria monocytogenes* and *E. coli* O157:H7. At the same time, FDA may inspect once every ten years soft cheeses or apple juice in which those same pathogens have been found. Some believe that it is inappropriate for separate agencies using different risk and inspection criteria to regulate the nation's food supply. These critics also think that the same or similar risk criteria should be used by all federal agencies to prevent microbial contamination on all foods.[20]

Others charge that safety cannot be properly regulated when food safety responsibility is placed in the hands of the same agency in charge also of promoting

---

[17]James T. O'Reilly, *Food and Drug Administration* (Colorado Springs, Colorado: Shepard's/McGraw-Hill, Inc., Oct. 1993).

[18]Edward L. Korwek, *1997 United States Biotechnology Regulations Handbook*, vol. 1, (Washington, D.C.:Food and Drug Law Institute, 1997), 112.

[19]Michael R. Taylor, "Preparing America's Food Safety System for the Twenty-First Century — Who is Responsible for What When it Comes to Meeting the Food Safety Challenges of the Consumer-Driven Global Economy?" in *Food and Drug Law Journal*, vol. 52, n.1, (Washington, D.C.:Food and Drug Law Institute, 1997) 13.

[20]Dr. Sanford Miller, Professor and Dean, Graduate School of Biomedical Sciences, The University of Texas Health Science Center at San Antonio, telephone conversation with the author, 17 September 1993, (210) 567–3709.

regulated products. Many think that an organization that promotes and subsidizes production agriculture and other consumer products should be separate from one that watches over food safety.

The meaning of "food safety" responsibilities continues to expand. Food safety functions of federal agencies have come to signify certain responsibilities regarding foods. The responsibilities were aptly defined in an FDA report to Congress:

> Under the foods program, FDA sets food standards; evaluates food additives and packaging for potential health hazards; conducts research to reduce food-borne disease to determine specific health impacts of hazardous substances in food and to develop methods for detecting them in foods; and maintains surveillance over foods through plant inspections, laboratory analyses, and legal action where necessary.[21]

USDA carries out similar functions for meats, poultry, and certain egg products.

Whether all food should be regulated by the same or different agencies is currently under debate. Some argue that a clearer direction to food safety policy could emerge if a single, independent agency were charged with administering all food safety programs. Others oppose forming a single agency, asserting that the various agencies with differing expertise strike a balance among divergent interests.

Recommendations for Changes in the Federal Organization of Food Safety Responsibilities

This report contains 21 separate sets of recommendations that have had a significant impact on the debate over whether the federal organization that ensures safe food needs to be changed. This debate has recurred over 48 years with long periods when little interest was expressed in changing the organization for federal food safety. The debate has been carried on by a range of different entities from major government bodies such as presidential commissions, agency commissions, congressional Members, the General Accounting Office (GAO), to interested parties or influential food policy experts.

The recommendations are grouped chronologically into four categories:

---

[21]Senate Committee on Agriculture, Rural Development, and Related Agencies, *Appropriation Bill, 1990*, 101st Cong., 2nd sess., 1989, S.Rept. 101-84, as found in Peter Barton Hutt and Richard A. Merrill, *Food and Drug Law: Cases and Materials*, 2nd ed. (Westbury, New York: The Foundation Press, Inc., 1991) 21.

- a separate, independent food safety agency or some modification of that idea;
- all food safety functions given to USDA;
- all food safety functions given to FDA;
- all food safety functions be given to the Consumer Product Safety Commission.

The recommendations described in this report were selected because each expresses a position on how the federal organization of food safety could be improved or changed. Each recommendation was acknowledged as contributing to the debate in later documents discussing changes in the organization for federal food safety. The gaps in the chronology represent the fluctuating nature of the debate. The recommendations listed also represent all the major official bodies that debated this issue in the last five decades.

No President or Congress has adopted these recommendations. However, the reports and publicity surrounding each set has added to the debate and helped define current food safety responsibilities. Eight sets of the recommendations would have created some type of independent federal entity for the regulation of food safety, with responsibility for all foods. Two would have given all responsibility to USDA, and 10 would have FDA reorganize and regulate the safety of all foods including meat and poultry. One would have the Consumer Product Safety Commission carry out all food safety functions. The most recent proposals appear to be evenly divided between giving food safety responsibility to a single, independent agency or to a reorganized FDA that links food safety explicitly to public health. Table 2, at the end of the report, summarizes in chronological order the selected sets of recommendations presented to Presidents and Congresses from 1949 to 1997 period.

Most of the reports or recommendations examine what are perceived to be five separate issues in food safety:

- Should food safety be considered to be a public health responsibility only or should it also be linked with research and development of new standards that not only protect consumers but also lead to the development and marketing of new products?
- Will the cost to the federal government increase or decrease if all activities related to regulating food are combined into a single food safety agency?
- By competing among each other for food safety resources, have agencies become more or less efficient in carrying out their food safety functions?
- If Congress and the Administration chose to create an independent food safety agency, should such an agency be independent of or located within the Public Health Service?
- Would U.S. consumers be better protected by having a uniform set of regulations and laws that covered all foods and were enforced by a single agency?

Some believe that one food safety agency could apply consistent and strong food standards that would assist in building public confidence in the federal system of food safety. Others argue that, although some consumers are very vocal in their distress with the current regulatory framework, it does provide some of the safest, most abundant, and least expensive food in the world.

Most believe that pressures for change will continue focusing mainly on streamlining policies for food, nutrition, and veterinary drug activities. There have always been threads that link the different food safety programs with those of production agriculture and nutrition research.

FOOD SAFETY UNDER A SINGLE, INDEPENDENT AGENCY

Popular Name and Date
White House Conference on Food, 1969.[22]

Description and Mission of Group Making Recommendations
President Nixon asked a large group of experts to meet and make recommendations on revising the federal regulatory policy for food and on certain aspects of food, nutrition, and health policy. He requested recommendations regarding administration and operations, community affairs, information, and education. The Conference was chaired by Dr. Jean Mayer, and the deputy chairman was James D. Grant.

Summary of Recommendations
The Conference recommended that there should be one federal regulatory policy with respect to safety, sanitation, identity, and labeling of foods. The Conference also recommended that the Secretary of Health, Education, and Welfare (HEW) issue an order establishing a separate interdepartmental coordinating committee on federal food regulatory policy with the aim of implementing national nutritional and health goals. The committee would be comprised of representatives of all federal departments and agencies having jurisdiction over safety, sanitation, identity, and labeling of any food. Within certain schedules, the committee should issue reports on the progress of reconciling all pertinent federal food policies and practices. The committee should initially consider the question of

---

[22]*White House Conference on Food, Nutrition, and Health, Final Report,* (Washington, D.C.: White House, 1969), 118–119.

whether a single federal regulatory agency for foods should be established, and particularly whether the jurisdiction of USDA over food products derived from or utilizing inspected meat and poultry should be transferred to HEW.

Dissenting views
Not Available

Popular Name and Date
GAO Food Inspection Report, 1970.[23]

Description and Mission of Group Making Recommendations

In a letter to the President of the Senate and the Speaker of the House of Representatives, the Comptroller General of the United States presented the results of a review of the roles of federal organizations involved in inspecting food. GAO's authority to conduct the review was contained in the Budget and Accounting Act of 1921 (31 U.S.C. 53); the Accounting and Auditing Act of 1950 (31 U.S.C. 67); and the authority of the Comptroller General to examine contractor's records as set forth in 10 U.S.C. 231(b).

Summary of Recommendations

Federal food inspection evolved from piecemeal legislation and regulations, designed to solve specific problems when they arose. The report claimed that current practice at the time did not clearly express an overall federal policy on food inspection. Many federal, state, and local organizations performed different parts of the food inspection process. Such a process led to some overlap in responsibility and caused dissatisfaction among members of the food industry. Some of the dissatisfaction related to inspections being made for different purposes and with varying intensity. The GAO recommended that the different agencies arrange agreements among themselves to use the skills and experience of each to establish clearer lines of responsibility, and to reduce overlap. The report did concede that those agreements would be time-consuming to arrange and difficult to administer.

Although the report did not specifically recommend consolidation, it criticized the overlapping inspection activities of USDA, FDA, and other federal agencies and the lack of consistency in their requirements, procedures, and concepts. GAO recommended that the Director, Bureau of the Budget, make a detailed evaluation of the federal food inspection system to see how to improve its administration and determine if it was feasible to consolidate some of the inspection efforts.

---

[23] General Accounting Office, *Need to Reassess Food Inspection Roles of Federal Organizations. Department of Agriculture, Department of Defense, Department of Health Education, and Welfare, Department of the Interior*, Rept. No. B-168966, 30 June 1970.

Dissenting views

Most of the federal agencies responsible for food inspections agreed to evaluate their separate functions. However, USDA's comments indicated that agency officials believed that GAO had not properly characterized certain USDA inspection functions. In its response letter, as published in the GAO report, it stated,

> Meat inspection, for example, is looked upon primarily as a program for consumer protection or benefit. This it is, but we believe it also facilitates interstate commerce in meats and enhances the market for farm animals sold for meat. Similarly meat grading, while it may be primarily looked upon as a program for facilitating marketing or dealing in meat, is recognized by consumers as a purchasing tool and, we believe as well, benefits the farmer by giving him added assurance of a return related to the quality of the animals sold. On the other hand, the consumer benefits from grading of grain are quite indirect. Performance standards are designed to be uniform whether the service is mandatory or voluntary. Thus procedures and regulations are geared to the particular need. The consumer's interests are expected to be recognized and protected in each case. It is the needs, and not whether the primary beneficiary is the producer, consumer, or industry that determines requirements and methods.

Popular Name and Date
Hearings on S. 3419, Consumer Safety Act of 1972.[24]

Description and Mission of Group Making Recommendations

Three committees of the Senate held hearings to discuss S. 3419, the Consumer Safety Act of 1972 and its proposal to restructure food safety responsibilities in the federal government. The Commerce Committee held a hearing on April 13, 1972. The Committee on Government Operations, Subcommittee on Executive Reorganization and Government Research held hearings on April 20, 21, May 2, 3, 1972. The Senate Labor and Public Welfare Committee, Subcommittee of Health held hearings on May 2, 3, 1972.

Summary of Recommendations

The report of the Senate Committee on Labor and Public Welfare stated that the purpose of S. 3419, the Consumer Safety Act of 1972, was to establish an independent agency to regulate foods, drugs, and consumer products. The bill

---

[24]Senate Committee on Commerce, *Consumer Safety Act of 1972*, 92nd Cong., 2nd sess., 1972, S.Rept. 92-749. Senate Committee on Government Operations, Subcommittee on Executive Reorganization and Government Research, *S.3419, The Consumer Safety Act of 1972*, 92nd Cong., 2nd sess., S.Rept. 92-2. Senate Committee on Labor and Public Welfare, *Food, Drug, and Consumer Product Safety Act of 1972*, 92nd Cong., 2nd sess., S.Rept. 92-835.

would have combined several different responsibilities under a single agency. For example, all FDA's authority to regulate foods and drugs would be transferred, as would the authority, at that time, of the Center for Disease Control over the licensing of certain clinical laboratories. The Department of Commerce and the Federal Trade Commission authority over flammable fabrics and refrigerator doors would be transferred as would USDA's authority over meat and poultry inspection and animal biological drugs. The purpose of this independent Consumer Safety Agency was to have been to protect consumers against unreasonable risk of injury from hazardous products. The independent agency would have had responsibility to set product safety standards for all consumer products representing unreasonable risk of injury or death.

S. 3419 became the Food, Drug, and Consumer Product Safety Act of 1972.[25] It passed the Senate on June 21. 1972. However, the House did not agree with the transfer of functions administered by FDA. In conference, legislators exempted all food, drugs, devices, and cosmetics as defined in the FFDCA from the jurisdiction of the new Consumer Product Safety Commission.

Dissenting Views

The Nixon Administration thought that the establishment of an independent consumer safety agency would prove to be regressive rather than progressive and opposed establishment of an independent "Consumer Safety Agency." On March 16, 1972, in a press release on S. 3419, Secretary of Health, Education, and Welfare Richardson stated,

> I think . . . that if the Food and Drug Administration is going to have any problems of digestion of new responsibilities, the problems would be multiplied several fold by the effort to create a new agency duplicating administrative authorities and having to seek scientific capabilities and resources that are already within the Food and Drug Administration. . . . It is . . . much greater if we build upon the experience and capabilities of the Food and Drug Administration, than if we start all over again through the creation of comparatively small, isolated outside body.[26]

---

[25]P.L. 92-573.

[26]Senate Committee on Commerce, *Consumer Safety Act of 1972*, 92nd Cong., 2nd sess., 1972, S.Rept. 92-749; Senate Committee on Government Operations, Subcommittee on Executive Reorganization and Government Research, *S.3419, The Consumer Safety Act of 1972*, 92nd Cong., 2nd sess., S.Rept. 92-2; Senate Committee on Labor and Public Welfare, *Food, Drug, and Consumer Product Safety Act of 1972*, 92nd Cong., 2nd sess., S.Rept. 92-835.

Popular Name and Year of Document
Ralph Nader Report, Sowing the Wind, 1972.[27]

Description and Mission of Group Making Recommendations

This report, sponsored by the Center for Study of Responsive Law, was conducted by an interdisciplinary task force of young professionals trained in law and science. Its members conducted research on a wide range of issues, from the fat and chemical content of hot dogs to the potential birth-defect hazards of pesticides. Ralph Nader wrote the introduction to the report. It had some influence on consumer opinion about certain food hazards.

Summary of Recommendations

The report found that food inspection "remains embarrassed by departmental conflicts of interest and overlapping jurisdictions in USDA and FDA." In its conclusions, the report recommended that meat inspection and chemical monitoring by USDA and FDA should be transferred to a new food safety agency where the goal of protecting public health would be consolidated. It also suggested that food inspection be included in the responsibilities of the independent "consumer safety agency" under consideration at the time in Congress.

Dissenting Views
Not Available

Popular Name and Date
GAO's Risk-Based Inspection Report, 1992.[28]

Description and Mission of Group Making Recommendations

GAO published this report in response to a request from the Honorable John D. Dingell, Chairman Subcommittee on Oversight and Investigations, House Committee on Energy and Commerce. GAO's mandate was to examine the consistency, efficiency, and effectiveness of the federal food safety inspection system.

Summary of Recommendations

GAO found that 12 agencies that were involved in food safety inspect similar foods posing similar risks at inconsistent frequencies and under different enforcement authorities. It also found long-standing problems whereby those agencies use

---

[27]Harrison Wellford, *Sowing the Wind: A Report from Ralph Nader's Center for Study of Responsive Law on Food Safety and the Chemical Harvest*, (New York: Grossman Publishers, 1972) 354.

[28]General Accounting Office, *Food Safety and Quality: Uniform, Risk-based Inspection System Needed to Ensure Safe Food Supply*, GAO/RCED-92-152, June 1992.

their inspection resources inefficiently and do not effectively coordinate with each other. GAO recommended that "Congress hold oversight hearings to evaluate options for revamping the federal food safety and quality system, including creating a single food safety agency responsible for administering a uniform set of food safety laws."

On October 8, 1997, a GAO division director advocated before the Senate Agriculture Committee that all federal food safety functions be assigned to a new agency. He stated that GAO "believes the existing federal food safety structure needs to be replaced with a uniform, risk-based inspection system under a single food safety agency. While some administrative actions can be taken to improve the system, the fundamental changes that are needed will require legislative action."[29]

Dissenting Views

DHHS officials responded to this GAO report by stating that there was no reason to believe that creating a new single agency would improve basic food safety. FDA, through DHHS, suggested that it could, without new legislation, formally establish regulations that could address the nature and extent of problems encountered by the food production industry; the food industry could be held accountable for self-regulation to an even greater degree; and a policy that compares risks could be established through regulation. The response implied that an independent agency was unnecessary. In addition, FDA claimed that the GAO report failed to analyze some major issues for the food industry such as whether the food industry needs uniformity in regulations by states and international harmonization of standards among countries; whether market promotion activities should be commingled with safety regulation; and whether the potential impact of new food technologies, both in producing and developing new and novel foods, would affect how regulations could ensure food safety.

Popular Name and Date
The Durenberger Food Safety Bill, 1993.[30]

Description and Mission of Group Making Recommendations

On August 3, 1993, Senator Durenberger introduced S. 1349, the Food Safety and Inspection Agency Act of 1993. It was referred to the Senate Committee on Governmental Affairs. There were no hearings on this bill.

---

[29]Robert A. Robinson, Director, Food and Agriculture Issues, RCED/GAO, "Food Safety: Fundamental Changes Needed to Improve the Nation's Food Safety System," statement for the record before the Senate Committee on Agriculture, Nutrition, and Forestry, 8 October 1997.

[30]S. 1349 was introduced by Senator Durenberger on 3 August 1993.

Summary of Recommendations

The act, if passed, would have placed all food safety and inspection activities in a single, independent agency that, with the guidance of a 15-person expert commission, would have set uniform risk-based inspection standards by which food safety could be ensured. It also would have established a state-federal communications network to educate consumers on potential microbial diseases.

Dissenting Views

Some critics claimed that the proposed bill did not clearly define what a uniform risk-based safety system was or how the existing two separate field-inspection systems would be organized. Also, critics claimed that this bill would have cost the federal government more to create a new agency than to transfer responsibility to an existing agency.

Popular Name and Date
The Torricelli/Bradley Food Safety Bill, 1994.[31]

Description and Mission of the Group Making Recommendations

The Katie O'Connell Safe Food Act (H.R. 3751) was introduced on January 26, 1994, by Representative Robert G. Torricelli. It was referred to the House Committees on Energy and Commerce and Agriculture. On February 1, 1994, it was referred to the Agriculture Subcommittees on Livestock, and Departmental Operations and Nutrition; and on February 24, 1994, it was referred to the Commerce Subcommittee on Health and the Environment. On August 2, 1994, Senator Bradley introduced the Katie O'Connell Safe Food Act (S. 2350); it was referred to the Senate Committee on Agriculture, Nutrition, and Forestry. No hearings were held on either bill. The bills received only a few cosponsors: three for H.R. 3751 and one for S. 2350.

Summary of Recommendations

The act, if it had passed, would have transferred responsibility for enforcing meat, poultry, and egg inspections from FSIS of USDA to an independent federal health agency called the Meat, Poultry and Eggs Inspection Agency. It would have created a position of director of meat, poultry, and eggs inspection and authorized 8 assistant directors. It also would have established an advisory commission made up of representatives from federal and state governments, industry, and the scientific community. This advisory commission would have recommended how the agency could improve inspection by using more technologically advanced techniques in meat, poultry, and egg product inspections.

---

[31]H.R. 3751 was introduced 26 January 1994; S.2350 was introduced 2 August 1994.

Dissenting Views

No dissenting views available, but the bill had few cosponsors.

Popular Name and Date

The Fazio-Durbin Food Safety Administration Bill, 1997.[32]

Description and Mission of Group Making Recommendations

In November 1997, Representative Vic Fazio and Senator Richard Durbin introduced identical bills, the Safe Food Act of 1997. On November 4, 1997, H.R. 2801 was referred to the Committees on Agriculture and Commerce and, on November 14, 1997, to the Subcommittee on Health and the Environment. S. 1465 was introduced on November 9, 1997, and referred to the Committee on Government Affairs. So far, there have been no hearings.

Summary of Recommendations

This act, if passed, would consolidate all federal food safety, labeling, and inspection programs into a new independent agency known as the Food Safety Administration (FSA). The new agency would be funded by transferring appropriated funds that are currently designated for food safety functions of four agencies (FDA, USDA, EPA, and National Marine Fisheries Service). According to supporters, the purpose of the new agency would be to replace an outdated, fragmented, and overlapping food safety system. Supporters also say that a single food safety agency could identify the most serious public health risks from specific food-borne pathogens. In addition, resources could be used to develop better testing methods, conduct risk assessments, and identify the most cost-effective interventions without regard to the type of food or bureaucratic "turf."

Dissenting Views

Critics believe that the time is not right for major reform of the current food safety system. Some resist the formation of a new agency because of fear that a whole new FSA would cause dislocation and upheaval. It could also mean that the current parent agencies would have to relinquish their budget authority and control over functions related to food safety. Most opponents to an independent agency advocate allowing the Clinton Administration's 1997 food safety initiatives to take effect. They await the Administration's reports to Congress as to whether these new policies reduce incidences of food-borne illnesses. Other critics claim that the proposed legislation does not define a new food safety mandate to be carried out, but only reorganizes food safety functions by moving the current functions to the new FSA. They argue that a new FSA could be hindered in setting priorities for

---

[32]H.R. 2801 was introduced 4 November 1997; S.1465 was introduced 9 November 1997.

food safety activities because the bills would not amend or change the basic food safety statutes that establish the policies on which the current food safety system is based. For example, the meat and poultry statutes require that a government inspector be in continuous attendance and the food and drug statute grants FDA the authority to act only when adulterated and/or misbranded foods are found in interstate commerce.

FOOD SAFETY UNDER THE
U.S. DEPARTMENT OF AGRICULTURE

Popular Name and Date
The Hoover Commission Report, May 20, 1949.[33]

Description and Mission of the Group Making Recommendations

Headed by Herbert Hoover, former President of the United States, the Commission on Organization of the Executive Branch of the Government was established in accordance with P. L.80-162, approved July 7, 1947. It was created by unanimous vote of Congress in July 1947, and submitted a series of reports to Congress. The Lodge-Brown Act, which brought the commission into being, conceived of its mission as being bipartisan. Therefore it had six members from each party. Four Commissioners each were chosen by the President of the Senate, the Speaker of the House of Representatives, and President Truman. The Commission members consisted of Herbert Hoover, Chairman; Dean Acheson, Vice Chair; Arthur S. Flemming; James Forrestal; George H. Mead; George D. Aikin; Joseph P. Kennedy; John L. McClellan; James K. Pollock; Clarence J. Brown; Carter Manasco; and James H. Rowe, Jr.

Summary of Recommendations

The commission recommended that all regulatory functions relating to food products be transferred to the Department of Agriculture and that those relating to other products be placed under a reorganized Drug Bureau administered by a public health agency. At the time, four agencies (Federal Security Agency, Federal Trade Commission, the Bureau of Internal Revenue in the Treasury Department, and USDA) exercised food regulatory functions, and some manufacturers had to comply with the regulations of more than one federal agency. The commission noted that many regulations related to food were once the responsibility of the

---

[33] *The Hoover Commission report on organization of the Executive Branch of the Government (1947–1949)*, Westport, CT: Greenwood Press, 1970).

Department of Agriculture. The commission found that, "their separation from other departmental activities [meaning USDA's activities]...creates great overlap and also confuses the public." With food inspections scattered among four government agencies, the commission argued that too many agencies had jurisdiction over food and drug products.

Dissenting views

Two of the commissioners, James K. Pollock, and James H. Rowe, Jr., disagreed with the recommendation to transfer the food regulatory activities of the FDA to USDA. They claimed that the purpose of the food provisions of the FFDCA was to protect the consumer. They advocated that a unified program under the FDA part of the Federal Security Agency should be kept together. They also stated that one food safety system under the FDA, that "safeguarded" consumers from a series of common problems, would accomplish that purpose. The common problems were characterized as "economic cheating (misleading and deceptive labels, substitution of cheaper ingredients, short weight); filth and other extraneous or obnoxious materials; harmful products or products containing harmful ingredients." The dissenting Commissioners also believed that splitting the regulatory functions of foods and drugs between two separate agencies would require two sets of laboratories and staffs working independently of each other and would limit the flexibility and economy of work assignments. These commissioners, the Committee on Medical Services, and the Brookings Institution recommended that the [food safety] function be continued as part of a reorganized public health service within the Federal Security Agency or its successor.

Popular Name and Date

Acts Restructuring Meat and Poultry Products Inspection:
Wholesome Meat Act of 1967 and the Poultry Products Act of 1968.[34]

Description and Mission of Group Making Recommendations

The Wholesome Meat Act of 1967[35] substantially revised the 1906 Meat Act. Soon afterwards, the Wholesome Poultry Act[36], signed on August 18, 1968, extended to poultry inspection many aspects of the meat inspection act approved in 1967. These acts were the result of a long debate over the differences in federal, state, and local meat inspections. The federal system continued to be responsible

---

[34]Vivian Wiser, "Part V: Meat and Poultry Inspection in the United States Department of Agriculture," in, *100 Years of Animal Health. 1884–1984*, eds.Vivian Wiser, Larry Mark, and H. Graham Purchase (Beltsville, MD: The Associates of the National Agricultural Library, 1986).

[35]P.L. 90-201.

[36]P.L. 90-492.

for meats moving in interstate commerce and international trade, whereas state and local authorities oversaw meats consumed in their own jurisdictions. Thus, the control over all meat products was mixed; some areas had rigid standards, and others had lax standards. From this background came a call for legislation setting common standards from various interested groups.

The Talmadge-Aiken Act of 1962 had provided for cooperation among federal and state agencies in regulating the marketing of agricultural products. However, few states took advantage of the authority to enter into broad cooperative agreements for meat inspection with USDA. Under the Talmadge-Aiken Act, the states were to establish "equal to" meat inspection systems. In 1967, President Johnson urged that the law be amended to provide greater protection to consumers and federal assistance to states in developing state inspection programs.

Summary of Recommendations

Both Acts required states to have meat and poultry inspection programs "at least equal in rigor to" federally-run programs (under APHIS), even though the state-inspected plants could still market their products only within the state. Under deadlines of December 1969 (meat) and August 1970 (poultry), states could receive federal matching funds to bring their programs up to federal safety and purity standards. One-year extensions could be granted under certain conditions. The Acts encouraged uniformity in the inspection systems and closed loopholes in various phases of the inspection program. Annual reports to Congress on operations and effectiveness of the inspection system were required.

Interest in restructuring the meat and poultry inspection systems had grown as certain Members of Congress became aware that some food additives were becoming a safety problem. Members received letters from constituents concerned about the presence of nitrosamine, a carcinogen, in bacon. Food processors added nitrite as a curing agent to pork, and that addition caused the formation of nitrosamine when the naturally occurring amine and nitrite combined. Consumers were also alarmed about meat safety when Canada prohibited meats from DES-treated animals (DES — Diethylstilbestrol — is a synthetic estrogenic drug) to be sold in its market. At the time, FDA considered banning its use altogether.

Dissenting views

There were charges that APHIS wanted the complete federalization of meat inspection. A number of representatives of the packing and processing industries joined others from some state agriculture departments opposing the new federal inspection programs. However, over time, the states dropped out of the meat inspection business because of its high cost. By 1976, APHIS inspectors monitored meat and poultry processing in 60% of the nation's plants.

FOOD SAFETY UNDER THE
FOOD AND DRUG ADMINISTRATION

Popular Name and Date
HEW Reorganization Directive of March 1968.[37]

Description and Mission of Group Making Recommendations

President Lyndon Johnson sent a message to Congress on March 4, 1968, with "Health Recommendations." Among the many proposals and recommendations was a directive to the Secretary of Health, Education, and Welfare to submit a "modern plan of organization to achieve the most efficient and economical operation of the health programs of the Federal Government." On March 13, 1968, the Secretary of Health, Education, and Welfare (HEW), Wilbur J. Cohen, announced his first step in carrying out the President's directive. He placed the FDA and the Public Health Service under the direction of Dr. Phillip R. Lee, the Assistant Secretary for Health and Scientific Affairs. The Commissioner of Food and Drugs would report directly to Dr. Lee, rather than to the Secretary. On June 14, 1968, Secretary Cohen's report to the President was made public and recommended the creation of a new Consumer Protection and Environmental Health Service (CPEHS) which would include FDA along with other agencies.

Summary of Recommendations

The rationale for making FDA a part of the newly created CPEHS was stated in the message from the Secretary to the President:

> The fact that similar or interacting contaminants manifest themselves in more than one type of environmental exposure argues strongly for focusing in a single agency the responsibility for identifying the hazards to health, developing and promulgating criteria and standards, and mounting programs that will promote compliance therewith. . . . Retention of a separate FDA relates to its history as a regulatory agency with an operational pattern historically different from that of the Public Health Service (PHS). The historic role of the FDA has been primarily one of policing industry to assure compliance with provisions of the FFDCA. . . . In the last two years, the FDA has markedly modified its policeman posture [with the food industry.]

The Secretary said that, with this new attitude and with states taking over most of the routine surveillance of industry practices, the justification of keeping FDA and PHS as separate agencies had disappeared.

---

[37]Wallace Janssen, "FDA Since 1962," in unpublished papers, *History of the Department of Health, Education and Welfare During the Presidency of Lyndon Baines Johnson, November 1963–January 1969*, kept in the FDA History Office by John Swan.

Dissenting views

In the 1968 reorganization Directive of the President, CPEHS was formed to deal with environmental problems, but it never received congressional authorization or appropriations. Other federal programs, funded at the time, contributed funding and positions. Dr. Winton Rankin, Deputy Commissioner of FDA reportedly commented: "We gave him [C.C. Johnson, Director of CPEHS] whatever bit of lip service we had to but didn't offer much cooperation. He finally went under." Dr. Rankin also said that he thought that if CPEHS succeeded, FDA would cease to exist.[38]

Popular Name and Date
The Malek Report, December 10, 1969.[39]

Description and Mission of Group Making Recommendations

On December 10, 1969, Frederick V. Malek, Deputy Undersecretary, Department of Health, Education, and Welfare became chairman of a Special Task Force on the Reorganization of the Consumer Protection Programs. The task force's report to Dr. Charles C. Edwards, FDA Commissioner, was called *Analysis and Recommendations: The Food and Drug Administration Organizational Review.* It contained an organizational and management study of the FDA. The report was delivered August 25, 1970.

Summary of Recommendations

The task force's report proposed a reorganization of FDA because of a growing concern over FDA's ability to carry out its consumer protection responsibilities. The report recommended that FDA become a separate health agency reporting to the Assistant Secretary for Health and Scientific Affairs, and a new Consumer Protection and Environmental Health Service be created separate from FDA. Within FDA, a new bureau for foods, pesticides, and product safety should be created along with a new drug bureau. Each should have full responsibility and authority from initial research to final regulatory action. The rationale was that the new Food Bureau could concentrate on its major product areas without jeopardizing other product areas and would create clearer lines of authority for FDA's compliance activities.

---

[38]Brannon, *Organizing and Reorganizing FDA,* 135–174.

[39]House Committee on Interstate and Foreign Commerce, Subcommittee on Commerce and Finance, *Hearings on the Consumer Product Safety Act,* 92nd Cong., 1st and 2nd sess., part 3, Nov. 1, 1971–Feb. 3, 1972, H.Rept. 92-61.

Dissenting Views
  Not Available

Popular Name and Date
Senate Governmental Affairs Report on Federal Regulation, 1977.[40]

Description and Mission of Group Making Recommendations
The Chairman of the Senate Committee on Governmental Affairs, Abraham Ribicoff, submitted *Study on Federal Regulation* to Walter F. Mondale, President of the Senate on December 21, 1977. The report was prepared under the authority of Senate Resolution 71, which authorized the Governmental Affairs Committee to conduct a study on various aspects of the federal regulatory process.

Summary of Recommendations
Senator Ribicoff hoped that the report would provide a basis for congressional action. The report recommended a transfer of USDA food regulatory functions to FDA. The report stated, "Divided responsibility for regulating food production has resulted in a regulatory program which is often duplicative, sometimes contradictory, undeniably costly, and unduly complex." The report asserted an urgent need to combine and rationalize the dual food regulation system that had existed over 70 years. "We believe the bifurcated food regulatory system should be unified in a single agency."

Dissenting Views
The proposal would have split employees located throughout the country (known as the field force) between the two administrations. USDA officials claimed that USDA's greatest strength was its network of field offices in operation throughout the country, as well as the experience and skills of its field staff. USDA officials were concerned that the transfer of USDA employees to another agency would weaken the network system.

---

[40]Senate Committee on Governmental Affairs, "V. Regulatory Organization" in *Study on Federal Regulation*, 95th Cong., 2d sess., December 1977, S.Rept. 95-91, 140.

Popular Name and Date
President Carter's 1978 Government Reorganization Project or White House Study (never released).[41]

Description and Mission of Group Making Recommendations
In February 1978, during testimony before the Appropriations Subcommittee on Agriculture, Rural Development and Related Agencies, chaired by Representative Whitten, spokespersons for the Carter Administration referred to the President's White House Study for Reorganization. Two of the most prominent officials were the Secretary of Agriculture, R. Bergland, and D. Angelotti, Administrator of the Food Safety and Quality Service (FSQS) (a precursor of FSIS).

Summary of Recommendations
The project recommended consolidation of all federal food regulatory functions. The final report did not resolve where the new organization would be located, although the HEW Secretary Joseph Califano suggested that FDA take over USDA's meat and poultry inspection and labeling duties. In 1977, USDA had formed the FSQS. Its mission was to enhance coordination among food inspection activities as well as food grading, certification and purchasing. USDA made clear that it had reorganized itself along functional lines, and, therefore, it did not believe consolidation of its food safety functions with FDA functions would be beneficial.

Dissenting Views
USDA Secretary Bergland countered Secretary Califano's suggestion with the idea that FDA food inspection authority be transferred to the new FSQS. Secretary Bergland stated, "The President's Reorganization Task Force is reviewing the desirability of combining FDA food activities, and USDA food safety and quality activities operations." In November 1977, HEW proposed that USDA's meat and poultry inspection activities and the women-infants-children program be consolidated within HEW. In February 1978, USDA proposed an alternative arrangement of functions. No final reorganization was initiated.

---

[41]House Committee on Appropriations, Subcommittee on Agriculture, Rural Development, and Related Agencies, *Hearings on Agriculture, Rural Development and Related Agencies Appropriations for 1979*, 95th Cong., 2nd sess., February 1978, 75 and 367–371.

Popular Name and Date
Lester Crawford, 1980.[42]

Description and Mission of Group Making Recommendations
From 1987 to 1991, Dr. Lester Crawford was the Administrator of USDA's Food Safety and Inspection Service. In a speech at the 1980 U.S. Animal Health Association annual meeting, he recommended that one agency would do a better job in formulating food regulatory policies.

Summary of Recommendations
Dr. Crawford stated, "Managerially unsound and duplicative systems of regulation will cause us all to still be spinning on our collective wheels decades from now." He suggested a number of alternatives: 1) consolidation of all food safety functions within DHHS; 2) transfer of FDA's Center of Food Safety and Applied Nutrition (CFSAN) and Center for Veterinary Medicine (CVM) to USDA; or 3) at least merge CFSAN with CVM.

Dissenting Views
Several food safety activists objected to moving all food safety responsibility to USDA, because USDA is not linked to the Public Health Service as is FDA. They argued that communication could be improved on food safety standards if all food safety agencies were affiliated with public health agencies such as the Centers for Disease Control and the National Institutes of Health.

Popular Name and Date
Dr. Sanford Miller, 1989.[43]

Description and Mission of Group Making Recommendations
Dr. Sanford Miller was the director of the Center for Food Safety and Applied Nutrition at FDA from 1978 to 1987. He is a national voice on public policy relating to nutrition and food sciences.

Summary of Recommendations
In discussing the underlying philosophical dynamic for the leading food safety agencies, which he believed has led to unnecessary controversies, Dr. Miller rec-

---

[42]Lester Crawford, "Critique of Animal Health Regulation," in *Proceedings of the 84th Annual Meeting*, (Washington, D.C., U.S. Animal Health Association, 1980.)

[43]Sanford Miller, "Quest for Safe Food: Knowledge and Wisdom," 1989 S. B. Hendricks Memorial Lecture of the USDA, ARS presented before the American Chemical Society, Miami Beach, Florida, 11 September 1989, (Washington:GPO, 1990), 11.

ommended that it was time to review the structure of food regulation in the United States. He suggested that it would be reasonable for the President and Congress to appoint a very senior level commission to review the requirements for an optimal food regulatory process and make recommendations. Dr. Miller stated, "The commission might very well conclude that the current setup is the best that we can devise, or it may propose a single agency, perhaps at the level of EPA."

Dissenting views
    Not Available

Popular Name and Date
The Edwards FDA Advisory Committee, May 1991.[44]

Description and Mission of Group Making Recommendations
    The committee was chaired by Dr. Charles C. Edwards, the former FDA Commissioner (1969–1973), and former Assistant Secretary for Health (1973–75). One of its members, Dr. David A. Kessler, later became the FDA Commissioner. The purpose of the committee was to examine FDA's mission, responsibility, and structure according to its legislative mandate, and to recommend how FDA could be strengthened to fulfill its mission. The committee was to provide advice accordingly to the Secretary of DHHS and to the Assistant Secretary for Health and did so in the *Final Report of the Advisory Committee on the Food and Drug Administration.*

Summary of Recommendations
    The Committee recommended that FDA be removed from the Public Health Service (PHS) and that the FDA Commissioner report directly to the Secretary of Health and Human Services. It also recommended that the Secretary of DHHS directly delegate to the Commissioner the authority to issue regulations implementing all the laws that FDA administers and to manage the daily operations of the Agency.
    The Food Policy Subcommittee of the Advisory Committee recommended that FDA move immediately to improve the Center for Food Safety and Applied Nutrition (CFSAN) management system, increase its resources, upgrade the development of its program planning, and delegate additional authority to the CFSAN director. It also recommended that the Commissioner establish one task force to ensure that FDA meet its nutrition labeling obligations and another to assist

---

[44]Department of Health and Human Services, *Advisory Committee on the Food and Drug Administration, Final Report,* May 1991, Charles C. Edwards, Chairman,, (Washington, 1991) iii–iv, 19–24.

CFSAN in resolving scientific and technical issues. It also said that it found no evidence to show that FDA's performance would improve if its human food responsibilities were combined with those of USDA. It recommended the establishment of a consistent approach to risk assessment among regulatory agencies responsible for food safety (FDA, EPA, and USDA), including for food derived from animals.

Dissenting Views

The Secretary of DHHS responded that the location in Public Health Service (PHS) was not the source of FDA problems. The Secretary contended that FDA gained from the close scientific interaction with other PHS agencies on issues such as AIDS epidemiology and research, pertussis vaccine, outbreaks of *Salmonella* Enteritidis, dental amalgam problems, and food safety issues.

Popular Name and Date
National Performance Review, September 1993.[45]

Description and Mission of Group Making Recommendations

Vice President Al Gore published his report of the National Performance Review (NPR) on September 7, 1993. He had been asked by President Clinton to undertake a 6-month study of the federal bureaucracy and make recommendations on how to create a government that works better and costs less.

Summary of Recommendations

The Review recommended that all federal food safety responsibilities be placed under the FDA.

Dissenting Views

A working group of government food safety officials advising the Vice-President's staff in preparing the NPR had recommended that an independent agency be created that would administer a science-based food safety system that would apply the same standards to all foods, thereby representing a more effective method of preventing food-borne illnesses. The working group also suggested that four policy initiatives were needed in conjunction with creating the new agency. The group suggested locating the new agency within the executive branch so that

---

[45] Al Gore, "From Red Tape to Results: Creating a Government That Works Better and Costs Less," in *Report of the National Performance Review,* (Washington, D.C., 7 September 1993), 101.

the congressional committees who would be responsible for oversight and the appropriation of its funds would be those "whose principal concerns are the health and economic welfare of this countries' citizens, and not those whose principal interests are in the economic welfare of the producers of food or the inspected food industries." The group also suggested that Congress should amend existing food safety laws to provide uniform regulatory authority that would be adequate to monitor and control food-borne health hazards at any point in the country's food production system. The group suggested that all food safety research functions be assigned to the single food safety agency. Finally, the group wanted the agency to fill each decision-making position with people who had appropriate scientific backgrounds.

None of those recommendations were in the final National Performance Review report. Some in Congress would have preferred that FSIS absorb all food and seafood inspection responsibilities. For example, House Speaker Thomas S. Foley said that, if USDA regulated all foods, the FDA would be free to concentrate on the safety of drugs.[46]

Popular Name and Date
Carol Tucker Foreman, Safe Food Coalition, October 6, 1993.[47]

Description and Mission of Group Making Recommendations
These recommendations, in the form of a press release issued by the Safe Food Coalition, reflect support for reorganizing food safety functions from the American Public Health Association, Center for Science in the Public Interest; Consumer Federation of America; Consumers Union; Food and Allied Service Trades AFL-CIO; Government Accountability Project; National Consumers League; Public Citizen; Public Voice for Food and Health Policy; United Food and Commodity Workers International Union. Ms. Foreman is a former Assistant Secretary of Agriculture.

Summary of Recommendations
The press release states that the Safe Food Coalition strongly endorses Vice President Gore's National Performance Review recommendation that would transfer USDA's meat and poultry inspection functions to FDA. The Coalition believes that the inspection of meat and poultry should be a public health program and

---

[46]Kenneth J. Cooper, "Hill Turf Fights May 'Reinvent' Gore Proposals," *Washington Post*, 13 September 1993, A19; Also see Rodney E. Leonard, "A Single Food Safety Agency," *Nutrition Week*, v. 23, September 1993, 2.

[47]Safe Food Coalition, "Safe Food Coalition Endorses Gore Proposal to Consolidate Food Safety Functions," Press Release and Letter to Members of the House, 6 October 1993, Ms. Joy Stevens, FDA/OLA, conversation with author, 2 September 1993.

should be within the responsibility of a public health agency. In supporting the consolidation of food safety functions within the FDA, the Coalition cited two concerns that they believed prevented USDA from effectively administering an adequate food safety inspection program. First, they believe that USDA knows more about animal health than human health, and second, that USDA cares more about promoting sales of agricultural products than it does about protecting consumers.

Dissenting Views

Giving the task of regulating meat and poultry to FDA would be similar to "the gnat swallowing the elephant," says a New York Times reporter, Marian Burros, in a newspaper article at the time.[48] FDA currently has about 1,042 full time equivalent (FTE) positions to do all types of inspection and to analyze food samples and other products, whereas FSIS of USDA has about 7,500 FTEs to inspect meat and poultry.

The types of inspections are somewhat different from one agency to the other. FDA staff pointed out that most FDA inspectors have extensive scientific training. FDA inspectors also make periodic inspections of food plants where they can take samples for laboratory analysis, check temperatures in canning processes, check machinery, and collect information in their evaluations to be able to support any regulatory action that may lead to a legal proceeding. FSIS staff explained that FSIS meat and poultry inspectors rely on constant and daily organoleptic inspection (based on sight, touch, or smell) of products as they flow by on the assembly line. FSIS inspectors can immediately condemn carcasses that do not pass standards. They also can take samples and send them for laboratory analysis, and inspect both the product and the paperwork connected with exports and imports.[49] In addition to the organoleptic approach, FSIS inspectors check each meat or poultry plant's Hazard Analysis and Critical Control Point (HACCP) plan and records. Every meat and poultry plant must implement, by the year 2000, a HACCP plan that identifies where hazards occur and what steps are needed to control those hazards.[50]

---

[48]Marian Burros, "Clinton Plan Would Move Meat and Poultry Inspections to FDA" *New York Times*, 13 September 1993, A18.

[49]Mrs. Joy Stevens, FDA/OLA, telephone conversation with author, 23 September 1993. Will Kerr, USDA/FSIS/BFPB, telephone conversation with author 24 September 1993.

[50]Congressional Research Service, *Food Safety Issues in the 105th Congress,*by Donna U. Vogt, IB98009, March 30, 1998; and *Meat and Poultry Inspection Issues,* by Jean Rawson, IB 95062, March 1998.

Popular Name and Date
**Hearings in Support of the Vice President's National Performance Review
Recommendations for Reinventing the Food Safety System, 1993–1994.[51]**

Description and Mission of Group Making Recommendations
A series of five hearings of two subcommittees of the House Committee on
Government Operations took place during both sessions of the 103rd Congress.
The Subcommittee on Human Resources and Intergovernmental Relations held
hearings on Nov. 4 and 19, 1993 (both were on USDA's progress in reforming
meat and poultry inspection); May 25, 1994 (review of FDA's food safety programs); Sept 28, 1994 (chemical residues and contaminants in food); and a joint
hearing with the Subcommittee on Information, Justice, Transportation, and Agriculture on June 16, 1994 (fresh versus frozen chickens and other issues involving
USDA's regulation of poultry products).

Summary of Recommendations
The hearing records contain thousands of pages of testimony and submitted
documents from hundreds of experts considering whether the current federal food
safety system is adequately protecting U.S. consumers; whether the existing system has a comprehensive federal food safety mission and objective that protects
the public's health; and whether Vice President Gore's National Performance
Review recommendation to consolidate all federal food safety programs within
FDA is warranted. Principally, most of the recommendations discussed the need to
revise the food safety system to monitor for microbiological pathogens in the food
supply and to prevent food-borne illnesses. Representative Edolphus Towns stated
in his opening remarks, "The current federal food safety system is not just fragmented; it is broken. The system is not designed to prevent food-borne disease...There is no question about it. USDA has known for over 20 years that its
inspection system cannot detect harmful microbes in meat and poultry, but did
absolutely nothing about it." Several witnesses also testified on the need to transfer
meat and poultry inspection functions to a "public health" agency because of the
perceived conflict in USDA's dual mission, agriculture production and consumer
protection.

Dissenting Views
USDA officials testified that they were implementing a "two track" approach
for reforming the meat and poultry safety system: first, to maximize the performance of the current inspection system; and second, to design, test, and implement a
regulatory program for the future. A key component of this approach was the
Pathogen Reduction Program/Hazard Analysis and Critical Control Point system

---

[51]House Committee on Government Operations, *Hearings on Reinventing the Federal Food Safety System*, 103rd Cong., 1st and 2nd sess, v. 1 and 2, 1995, Joint Committee
Print.

aimed at reducing the likelihood of harmful microorganisms that could enter the food system anywhere in the production, distribution, and consumption chain. USDA officials and representatives from state agriculture and health departments testified that there was no need to reorganize food safety activities because, in carrying out food safety inspections and other activities, they were ensuring already that the foods under their jurisdictions were safe.

FOOD SAFETY UNDER THE CONSUMER PRODUCT SAFETY COMMISSION

Popular Name
The Metzenbaum Bill, 1993.[52]

Description and Mission of Group Making Recommendations
The Food Safety Reform Act of 1993 (S. 1750) was introduced on November 20, 1993, by Senator Metzenbaum and was referred to the Senate Committee on Governmental Affairs. S. 1750 had no cosponsors.

Summary of Recommendations
The act would have transferred to the Consumer Product Safety Commission (CPSC) all food safety and inspection functions of the USDA and the Departments of the Interior and Commerce, FDA, and EPA. It would have established the position of "Executive Director of Food Safety" in the CPSC, which would be charged with preparing and submitting to the appropriate congressional committees a plan for a nationwide food safety database and the implementation of food inspection techniques. The plan would include hazard analysis of critical control points, rapid pathogen detection, trace-back technology, food irradiation, and other necessary techniques. The purpose of this bill would have been to centralize responsibility for the management of all federal food safety activities into one existing agency to lessen the cost on the federal budget.
Dissenting Views
Not Available

---

[52]S. 1750 was introduced 20 November 1993.

Table 2. Recommendations for Changes in the Federal Organization of Food Safety Responsibilities, 1949–1997 (In chronological order)

Name and Source	Proposed Changes in Organization
1949 The Hoover Commission Report. U.S. Commission on Organization of the Executive Branch of the Government (1947–1949). May 20, 1949. Westport, CT:Greenwood Press, 1970.	Recommended that all regulatory functions relating to food products to protect the consumer be transferred to USDA and that those relating to other products be placed under a reorganized Drug Bureau administered by the public health agency.
1968 Department of Health, Education, and Welfare Reorganization Directive of March. Found in: Janssen, Wallace. FDA Since 1962. Vol. 1. Unpublished papers entitled History of the Department of Health, Education and Welfare During the Presidency of Lyndon Baines Johnson. November 1963–January 1969.	Placed FDA under the Public Health Service and in July 1968 made FDA a part of the newly created Consumer Protection and Environmental Health Service (CPEHS). FDA received resources devoted to pesticides, shellfish, product safety, and poison control from other Public Health agencies. FDA then began to operate under the Public Health Service Act.
1967–68 Acts Restructuring of Meat and Poultry Inspection: Wholesome Meat Act of 1967, and the Poultry Products Act of 1968. U.S. Department of Agriculture. Economic Research Service. National Economy and History Branch. Agriculture and Rural History Branch. Unpublished chapters from forthcoming history of the Food Safety and Inspection Service.	Both required states to have meat and poultry inspections programs "at least equal in rigor to" federally run programs (under APHIS), even though the state-inspected plants could still only market their products within the state. Under deadlines of December 1969 (meat) and August 1970 (poultry), states could receive federal matching funds to bring their programs up to federal safety and purity standards. One-year extensions were to be granted under certain conditions.
1969 White House Conference on Food, Nutrition, and Health. Final Report. Washington, D.C. 1969.	Recommended that there should be one federal regulatory policy with respect to safety, sanitation, identity, and labeling of foods.

Table 2. Recommendations for Changes in the Federal Organization of Food Safety Responsibilities, 1949–1997, cont.

1969 Malek Report. House Committee on Interstate and Foreign Commerce. Subcommittee on Commerce and Finance. Consumer Product Safety Act. Hearings, 92nd Congress, 2nd sess. Part 3, Nov. 1, 1971–Feb. 3, 1972. Serial No. 92-61. Washington, U.S. Govt. Print. Off., 1972.	Recommended that a new Consumer Protection and Environmental Health Service be created, separate from FDA, with FDA becoming a major health agency reporting to the Assistance Sec. for Health and Scientific Affairs. Within FDA, a new Bureau of Foods, Pesticides, and Product Safety and a Bureau of Drugs would be created, each with full responsibility and authority for all activities from initial research to final regulatory action.
1970 General Accounting Office, Need to Reassess Food Inspection Roles of Federal Organizations. Department of Agriculture, Department of Defense, Department of Health Education, and Welfare, Department of the Interior. Report to the Congress by the Comptroller General of the United States. Rept. No. B-168966. June 30, 1970.	Did not specifically recommend consolidation, but criticized the overlapping inspection activities among USDA, FDA, and other federal agencies. Instead, it recommended that the Director, Bureau of the Budget, make a detailed evaluation of the federal food inspection system to see how to improve its administration and determine if it was feasible to consolidate some of the inspections.
1972 Ralph Nader Report. Wellford, Harrison. Sowing the Wind: A Report from Ralph Nader's Center for Study of Responsive Law on Food Safety and the Chemical Harvest. (New York: Grossman Publishers, 1972), 354.	Found that food inspection "remains embarrassed by departmental conflicts of interest and overlapping jurisdictions in USDA and FDA." In its conclusions, the report recommended that meat inspection and chemical monitoring by USDA and the food inspection functions of FDA be transferred to a new food safety agency to improve the likelihood of protecting the public health.

Table 2. Recommendations for Changes in the Federal Organization of Food Safety Responsibilities, 1949–1997, cont.

1972 Hearings before the U.S. Senate on S. 3419. Senate Committee on Commerce, Consumer Safety Act of 1972, 92nd Cong., 2nd sess., 1972, S.Rept. 92-749. Senate Committee on Government Operations, Subcommittee on Executive Reorganization and Government Research, S.3419, The Consumer Safety Act of 1972, 92nd Cong., 2nd sess., S.Rept. 92-2. Senate Committee on Labor and Public Welfare, Food, Drug, and Consumer Product Safety Act of 1972, 92nd Cong., 2nd sess., S.Rept. 92-835.	The purpose of S. 3419, Consumer Safety Act of 1972, was to establish an independent agency to regulate foods, drugs, and consumer products. The bill would have combined under a single agency, a number of different responsibilities. The purpose of this independent Consumer Safety Agency was to have been to protect consumers against unreasonable risk of injury from hazardous products. The independent agency would have had responsibility to set product safety standards for all consumer products representing unreasonable risk of injury or death. S. 3419 became the umbrella legislation and was called the Food, Drug, and Consumer Product Safety Act of 1972. It passed the Senate on June 21. 1972.
1977, Senate Committee on Governmental Affairs Report. U.S. Congress. Senate. Committee on Governmental Affairs. Study on Federal Regulation. Senate Document No. 95-91, 95th Cong., 2d sess. vol. V. Regulatory Organization. December 1977. p. 140.	Recommended a transfer of USDA food regulatory functions to FDA.
1978 President Carter's Government Reorganization Project or White House Study (never released). U.S. Congress. House Committee on Appropriations, Subcommittee on Agriculture, Rural Development, and Related Agencies. Agriculture, Rural Development and Related Agencies Appropriations for 1979. Hearings, Parts 1 and 4, Feb., 1978. Washington, D.C., U.S. Govt. Print. Off., 1978. p. 75 (pt.1), p. 367–371 (pt. 4).	Recommended consolidation of all food regulatory functions of FDA.
1980 Lester Crawford Speech. Crawford, Dr. Lester. Critique of Animal Health Regulation. Proceedings of the 84th Annual Meeting. Washington, D.C., U.S. Animal Health Association, 1980.	Suggested consolidation of all food safety functions within DHHS, transfer of FDA's divisions of Center of Food Safety and Applied Nutrition (CFSAN) and Center for Veterinary Medicine (CVM)to USDA, or at least merge CFSAN with CVM.

Table 2. Recommendations for Changes in the Federal Organization of Food Safety Responsibilities, 1949–1997, cont.

1989 Dr. Sanford Miller. Quest for Safe Food: Knowledge and Wisdom. 1989 S. B. Hendricks Memorial Lecture presented by Dr. Sanford A. Miller by USDA, ARS before the American Chemical Society, Miami Beach, Florida. September 11, 1989. U.S. Department of Agriculture. Agricultural Research Service. Washington, D.C., U.S. Govt. Print. Off., 1990. p. 11.

Recommended that a special commission be set up to make recommendations on the optimal food safety regulatory process which may be a single agency.

1991 The Edwards Committee Report. U.S. Dept. of Health and Human Services. Advisory Committee on the Food and Drug Administration. Final Report. Charles C. Edwards, Chairman. May 1991. Washington, D.C., 1991. p. iii–iv, 19–24.

Recommended that FDA be removed from the Public Health Service (PHS) and the FDA Commissioner report directly to the Secretary of Health and Human Services

1992 Risk-Based Food Safety Inspection. U.S. General Accounting Office. Food Safety and Quality: Uniform, Risk-based Inspection system Needed to Ensure Safe Food Supply. GAO/RCED-92-152, June 1992.

Recommended that Congress hold oversight hearings to evaluate options for revamping the federal food safety and quality system, including creating a single food safety agency responsible for administering a uniform set of food safety laws.

1993 S. 1349, Food Safety and Inspection Agency Act was introduced by Senator Durenberger and referred to the Senate Committee on Governmental Affairs, August 3, 1993.

Would have placed all food safety and inspection activities in a single, independent agency which would, with the guidance of a 15-person expert commission, set uniform risk-based inspection standards by which food safety would be ensured. In addition, it would have established a state-federal communications network to educate consumers on potential microbial diseases.

1993. National Performance Review. Gore, Al. From Red Tape to Results: Creating a Government that Works Better and Costs Less. Report of the National Performance Review. Washington, D.C. September 7, 1993, 101.

Recommended consolidating all federal food safety responsibilities under the FDA.

Table 2. Recommendations for Changes in the Federal Organization of Food Safety Responsibilities, 1949–1997, cont.

1993. Carol Tucker Foreman and the Safe Food Coalition, "Safe Food Coalition Endorses Gore Proposal to Consolidate Food Safety Functions," Press Release and Letter to Members of the House, 6 October 1993 in which they strongly supported the National Performance Review recommendation to move the food safety function of inspection of meat and poultry to the FDA. The Coalition is composed of members of the from the American Public Health Association; Center for Science in the Public Interest; Consumer Federation of America; Consumers Union; Food and Allied Service Trades, AFL-CIO; Government Accountability Project; National Consumers League; Public Citizen; Public Voice for Food and Health Policy; United Food and Commercial Workers International Union.

States that the Safe Food Coalition strongly endorses Vice President Gore's National Performance Review recommendation that would transfer USDA's meat and poultry inspection functions to FDA. The Coalition believes that the inspection of meat and poultry should be a public health program and should be within the responsibility of a public health agency. In supporting the consolidation of food safety functions within the FDA, the Coalition cited two concerns that they believed prevented USDA from effectively administering an adequate food safety inspection program. First, they believe that USDA knows more about animal health than human health, and second, that USDA cares more about promoting sales of agricultural products than it does about protecting consumers.

1993 and 1994 Hearings in Support of the Vice President's National Performance Review Recommendations for Reinventing the Food Safety System. House Committee on Government Operations, Hearings, *Reinventing the Federal Food Safety System*, 103rd Cong., 1st and 2nd Sess., Volume 1 and 2. Washington, D.C.:GPO, 1995.

Hearing experts discussed whether the current federal food safety system was adequately protecting U.S. consumers, whether the existing system has a comprehensive federal food safety mission and objective that can protect the public health, and whether Vice President Gore's National Performance Review recommendation to consolidate all federal food safety programs within FDA is warranted.

1993 The Food Safety Reform Act (S. 1750) was introduced on November 20, 1993 by Senator Metzenbaum and referred to the Senate Committee on Governmental Affairs.

Would have transferred to the Consumer Product Safety Commission (CPSC) all food safety and inspection functions of the USDA, and the Departments of the Interior and Commerce, FDA, and EPA.

Table 2. Recommendations for Changes in the Federal Organization of Food Safety Responsibilities, 1949–1997, cont.

1994 The Katie O'Connell Safe Food Act (H.R. 3751) was introduced on January 26, 1994 by Representative Robert G. Torricelli; it was referred to the House Committees on Energy and Commerce and Agriculture. On February 24, 1994, it was referred to the Commerce Subcommittee on Health and the Environment; and on Feb. 1, 1994 it was referred to the Agriculture Subcommittees on Livestock, and Departmental Operations and Nutrition. On August 2, 1994, Senator Bradley introduced the Katie O'Connell Safe Food Act (S. 2350); it was referred to the Senate Committee on Agriculture, Nutrition, and Forestry.	Would have transferred responsibility for enforcing meat, poultry, and egg inspections from FSIS of USDA to an independent federal health agency entitled the Meat, Poultry and Eggs Inspection Agency.
1997 The Safe Food Act of 1997 (H.R. 2801/S. 1465). Rep. Vic Fazio and Sen. Richard Durbin introduced identical bills. On Nov. 4, 1997, H.R. 2801 was referred to the Committees on Agriculture and Commerce and on Nov. 14, 1997, H.R. 2801 was referred to the Subcommittee on Health and the Environment. S. 1465 was introduced on Nov. 9, 1997, and referred to the Committee on Government Affairs.	Would consolidate all federal food safety, labeling, and inspection programs into a new single, independent agency known as the Food Safety Administration (FSA). The purpose of the agency would be to identify the most serious public health risks from specific food borne pathogens and use resources to develop improved testing methods, conduct risk assessments, and identify the most cost-effective interventions without regard to the type of food or bureaucratic "turf."

C

Food Safety from Farm to Table: A National Food-Safety Initiative[*]

A Report to the President
May 1997

Executive Summary

---

[*]SOURCE: Copied from internet location:**http://vm.cfsan.fda.gov/~dms/fsreport.html**.

TABLE OF CONTENTS

Executive Summary

A New Interagency Strategy to Prevent Foodborne Disease

Foodborne Illness: A Significant Public-Health Problem
    Sources of Foodborne Contamination
    The Current System for Protecting Food
    The Food-Safety System Must Be Prepared for the 21st Century
    Immediate Actions to Improve Food Safety
    A New Early-Warning System for Foodborne Disease Surveillance
    Interstate Outbreak Containment and Response Coordination
    Risk Assessment
    Research
    Improving Inspections and Compliance
    Education
    A Blueprint for a Better Food-Safety System

Appendix A: Budget Request for Food-Safety Initiative Activities: FY98

Appendix B: Microbial Pathogens

---

* This appendix reproduces only the Executive Summary of *Food Safety from Farm to Table*. The contents of the entire report, from which the Executive Summary has been extracted are given here for the reader information—

EXECUTIVE SUMMARY

While the American food supply is among the safest in the world, there are still millions of Americans stricken by illness every year caused by the food they consume, and some 9,000 a year—mostly the very young and elderly—die as a result. The threats are numerous and varied, ranging from *Escherichia coli* (*E. coli*) O157:H7 in meat and apple juice, to *Salmonella* in eggs and on vegetables, to *Cyclospora* on fruit, to *Cryptosporidium* in drinking water—and most recently, to hepatitis A virus in frozen strawberries.

In his January 25, 1997 radio address, President Clinton announced he would request $43.2 million in his 1998 budget to fund a nationwide early-warning system for foodborne illness, increase seafood safety inspections, and expand food-safety research, training, and education. The President also directed three Cabinet members—the Secretary of Agriculture, the Secretary of Health and Human Services, and the Administrator of the Environmental Protection Agency—to identify specific steps to improve the safety of the food supply. He directed them to consult with consumers, producers, industry, states, universities, and the public, and to report back to him in 90 days. This report responds to the President's request and outlines a comprehensive new initiative to improve the safety of the nation's food supply.

The goal of this initiative is to further reduce the incidence of foodborne illness to the greatest extent feasible. The recommendations presented in this report are based on the public-health principles that the public and private sectors should identify and take preventive measures to reduce risk of illness, should focus our efforts on hazards that present the greatest risk, and should make the best use of public and private resources. The initiative also seeks to further collaboration between public and private organizations and to improve coordination within the government as we work toward our common goal of improving the safety of the nation's food supply.

Six agencies in the federal government have primary responsibility for food safety: two agencies under the Department of Health and Human Services (HHS)—the Food and Drug Administration (FDA) and the Centers for Disease Control and Prevention (CDC); three agencies under the Department of Agriculture (USDA)—the Food Safety and Inspection Service (FSIS), the Agricultural Research Service (ARS), and the Cooperative State Research, Education, and Extension Service (CSREES); and the Environmental Protection Agency (EPA). Over the last 90 days, these agencies have worked with the many constituencies interested in food safety to identify the greatest public-health risks and design strategies to reduce these risks. USDA, FDA, CDC, and EPA have worked to build consensus and to identify opportunities to better use their collective resources and expertise, and to strengthen partnerships with private organizations. As directed by the President, the agencies have explored ways to strengthen systems of coordination, surveillance, inspections, research, risk assessment, and education.

This report presents the results of that consultative process. It outlines steps USDA, HHS, and EPA will take this year to reduce foodborne illness, and spells out in greater detail how agencies will use the $43.2 million in new funds requested for fiscal year 1998. It also identifies issues the agencies plan to consider further through a public planning process.

The actions in this report build on previous Administration steps to modernize our food-safety programs and respond to emerging challenges. As part of the Vice President's National Performance Review (NPR), the agencies have encouraged the widespread adoption of preventive controls. Specifically, the NPR report urged implementation of Hazard Analysis and Critical Control Point (HACCP) systems to ensure food manufacturers identify points where contamination is likely to occur and implement process controls to prevent it. Under HACCP-based regulatory programs there is a clear delineation of responsibilities between industry and regulatory agencies: Industry has the primary responsibility for the safety of the food it produces and distributes; the government's principle role is to verify that industry is carrying out its responsibility, and to initiate appropriate regulatory action if necessary.

The Administration has put in place science-based HACCP regulatory programs for seafood, meat, and poultry. In late 1995, the Administration issued new rules to ensure seafood safety. In July 1996, President Clinton announced new regulations to modernize the nation's meat and poultry inspection system. The Early-Warning System the President announced in January will gather critical scientific data to further improve these prevention systems. Additional actions outlined in this report will encourage the use of HACCP principles throughout the food industry.

The need for further action is clear. Our understanding of many pathogens and how they contaminate food is limited; for some contaminants, we do not know how much must be present in food for there to be a risk of illness; for others, we do not have the ability to detect their presence in foods. The public-health system in this country has had a limited ability to identify and track the causes of foodborne illness; and federal, state, and local food-safety agencies need to improve coordination for more efficient and effective response to outbreaks of illness. Resource constraints increasingly limit the ability of federal and state agencies to inspect food processing facilities (e.g., years can go by before some plants receive a federal inspection.) Increasing quantities of imported foods flow into this country daily with limited scrutiny. Some food processors, restauranteurs, food-service workers, supermarket managers, and consumers are unaware of how to protect food from the threat of foodborne contaminants. These and other deficiencies will be addressed by key Administration actions outlined in this report and described below.

Enhance Surveillance and Build an Early-Warning System

As the President announced in January, the Administration will build a new national early-warning system to help detect and respond to outbreaks of foodborne illness earlier, and to give us the data we need to prevent future outbreaks. For example, with FY98 funds, the Administration will:

Enhance Surveillance. The Administration will expand from five to eight the number of FoodNet active surveillance sentinel sites. Personnel at these sentinel sites actively look for foodborne diseases. Existing sites are in Oregon, Northern California, Minnesota, Connecticut, and metropolitan Atlanta. New sites will be in New York and in Maryland, with an eighth site to be identified. CDC will also increase surveillance activities for certain specific diseases. For example, CDC will begin a case-control study of hepatitis A to determine the proportion of cases due to food contamination, FDA will strengthen surveillance for Vibrio in Gulf Coast oysters, and CDC will strengthen surveillance for *Vibrio* in people.

Equip FoodNet sites and other state health departments with state-of-the-art technology, including DNA fingerprinting, to identifythe source of infectious agents and with additional epidemiologistsand food-safety scientists to trace outbreaks to their source.

Create a national electronic network for rapid fingerprint comparison. CDC will equip the sentinel sites and other state health departmentswith DNA fingerprinting technology, and will link states together to allow the rapid sharing of information and to quickly determinewhether outbreaks in different states have a common source.

Improve Responses to Foodborne Outbreaks

At the federal level, four agencies are charged with responding to outbreaks of foodborne and waterborne illness: CDC, FDA, FSIS, and EPA. States and many local governments with widely varying expertise and resources also share responsibility for outbreak response. The current system does not assure a well-coordinated, rapid response to interstate outbreaks. To ensure a rapid and appropriate response, with FY98 funds, agencies will:

Establish an Intergovernmental Foodborne Outbreak Response Coordinating Group. Federal agencies will form an intergovernmental group, the Foodborne Outbreak Response Coordinating Group, to improve the approach to interstate outbreaks of foodborne illness. This group will provide for appropriate participation by representatives of stateand local agencies charged with responding to outbreaks of foodborne illness. It will also review ways to more effectively involve theappropriate state agencies when there is a foodborne outbreak.

Strengthen the infrastructure for surveillance and coordination at state health departments. CDC, EPA, FDA, and FSIS will assess andcatalogue available state resources, provide financial and technicalsupport for foodborne-disease-surveillance programs, and otherassistance to better investigate foodborne-disease outbreaks.

Improve Risk Assessment

Risk assessment is the process of determining the likelihood that exposure to a hazard, such as a foodborne pathogen, will result in harm or disease. Risk-assessment methods help characterize the nature and size of risks to human health associated with foodborne hazards and assist regulators in making decisions about where in the food chain to allocate resources to control those hazards. To improve risk-assessment capabilities, with FY98 funds, the agencies will:

Establish an interagency risk assessment consortium to coordinate and guide overarching federal risk-assessment research related to food safety.

Develop better data and modeling techniques to assess exposure to microbial contaminants, and simulate microbial variability from farm to table. Such techniques will help scientists estimate, for example, how many bacteria are likely to be present on a food at the point that it is eaten (the end of the food chain), given an initial level of bacteria on that food as it entered the food chain.

Develop New Research Methods

Today, many pathogens in food or animal feed cannot be identified. Other pathogens have developed resistance to time-tested controls such as heat and refrigeration. With FY98 funds, the agencies will focus research immediately to:

Develop rapid, cost-effective tests for the presence in foods of pathogens such as *Salmonella, Cryptosporidium, E. coli* O157:H7, and hepatitis A virus in a variety of foods, especially foods already associated with foodborne illness.

Enhance understanding of how pathogens become resistant to food-preservation techniques and antibiotics.

Develop technologies for prevention and control of pathogens, such as by developing new methods of decontamination of meat, poultry, seafood, fresh produce, and eggs.

Improve Inspections and Compliance

With FY98 funds, the agencies will pursue several strategies to increase inspections for higher-risk foods; the agencies will, among other things:

Implement seafood HACCP. FDA will add seafood inspectors to implement new seafood HACCP regulations, and will work with the Commerce Department to integrate Commerce's voluntary seafood-inspection program with FDA's program.

Propose preventive measures for fresh fruit and vegetable juices. Based on the best science available, FDA will propose appropriate regulatory and non-regulatory options, including HACCP, for the manufacture of fruit and vegetable juice products.

Propose preventive measures for egg products. Based on the best science available, FSIS will propose appropriate regulatory and non-regulatory options, including HACCP, for egg products.

Identify preventive measures to address public-health problems associated with produce such as those recently associated with hepatitis A virus in frozen strawberries and *E. coli* O157:H7 on lettuce. These measures will be identified through a comprehensive review of current production and food-safety programs including inspection, sampling, and analytical methods.

Improve coverage of imported foods. FDA will develop additional mutual recognition agreements (MRAs) with trading partners, initiate a federal-state communication system covering imported foods, and FDA and FSIS will provide technical assistance to countries whose products are implicated in a foodborne illness.

Further Food-Safety Education

Foodborne illness remains prevalent throughout the United States, in part because food preparers and handlers at each point of the food chain are not fully informed of risks and related safe-handling practices. Understanding and practicing proper food-safety techniques, such as thoroughly washing hands and cooking foods to proper temperatures, could significantly reduce foodborne illness. The Administration—working in partnership with the private sector—will use FY98 funds to, among other things:

Establish a Public-Private Partnership for Food-Safety Education. FDA, USDA, CDC, and the Department of Education will work with the food industry, consumer groups and the states to launch a food-safety public awareness and education campaign. The Partnership will develop, disseminate, and evaluate a single food-safety slogan and several standard messages. Industry has pledged $500,000 to date to support the partnership's activities and plans to raise additional funds.

Educate professionals and high-risk groups. Agencies will better educate physicians to diagnose and treat foodborne illness; strengthen efforts to educate producers, veterinarians, and state and local regulators about proper animal drug use and HACCP principles; and work with the Partnership to better train retail- and food-service workers in safe handling practices and to inform high-risk groups about how to avoid foodborne illness, e.g., in people with liver disease, illness that may be caused by consuming raw oysters containing *Vibrio vulnificus*.

Enhance federal-state inspection partnerships. New federal-state partnerships focused on coordinating inspection coverage (particularly between FDA and the states) will be undertaken, in an important step towards ensuring the effectiveness of HACCP and ensuring that the highest-risk food plants are inspected at least once per year.

Continue the Long-Range Planning Process

Through this initiative, and through previous activities, HHS, USDA, and EPA have laid the groundwork for a strategic planning effort. There is a broad recognition of the need to carefully implement the initiative's programs, and to consider how to apply preventive measures in other areas of concern. A strategic-planning effort is needed to build on this common ground, and to tackle some of the difficult public-health, resource, and management questions facing federal food-safety agencies. The federal food-safety agencies are committed to continuing to meet with stakeholders, ultimately to produce a strategic plan for improving the food-safety system.

D

Workshop Presentation Summaries and Workshop Agenda

The following pages summarize in the committee's words the key points from the presentations given at the public workshop on April 29–30, 1998 (see agenda at end of summary). The workshop was organized in three phases: first, two speakers presented information concerning international food safety systems and organizational strategies to the committee. The second phase was organized to assist the committee in gathering feedback from various stakeholders concerning the current food safety system and changes that would lead to a more effective system. The committee asked these presenters to respond in writing and provide oral testimony to the following questions:

- What works well in the current US food safety system?
- What changes would lead to a more effective food safety system?
- What types of changes would be detrimental to an effective food system?

The third phase was designed to provide an opportunity for public comment regarding the US food safety system.

Copies of the written testimonies submitted to the committee by workshop presenters are available from the National Academy of Sciences' (NAS) public information file. Information on accessing these documents is available from the NAS website at **http://www.nas.edu.**

PHASE I:

International Perspectives for Ensuring Safe Food (Ian Munro, CanTox, Inc.)
- A disassociation of regulatory and inspection activities may be evolving in international systems that are undergoing change.
- In Canada, the regulatory component is divided among agriculture, health, and environmental divisions. A fee for service system is being utilized, which needs to be assessed as to its overall budget impact.
- Finland has a unique system. It is a small country with responsibilities distributed between political and technical cabinets.
- In New Zealand, inspection is privatized.
- It is difficult to determine whether changes in food safety systems in other countries have improved the situation, because there are no benchmarks from which to measure improvement or progress.
- Most countries have emphasized the use of external expertise in developing effective food safety systems.

Organizational Strategies (J. Clarence [Terry] Davies, Resources for the Future)
- It is possible that changes in the current US food safety system could result in the worst of both worlds.
- EPA was organized partly on topic and function. Their organizational plan was not entirely implemented.
- Localizing efforts in one agency may reduce priority for the issues in other agencies; however, focus by one agency reduces duplication.
- Combining efforts in one agency will also increase visibility of the issue. Since the formation of the EPA, environmental activities have increased.
- Strong leadership is critical.
- It is important to know whether changes in organization are being recommended based on function or based on cost efficiency. Reasons for changes must be clearly explained.
- Often changes suggested to increase effectiveness may not result in cost savings.
- It will be difficult to develop new approaches and attitudes without breaking up the old system.
- The separation of regulatory efforts from research efforts is likely to lead to better science.

PHASE 2:   PANEL PRESENTATIONS

Food Producers Panel
- *Animal Agriculture Coalition (Gary Weber)*
    - supports HACCP, partnerships, and the use of science and technology; and
    - no need for more regulation to solve problems.

- *The National Council of Farmer Cooperatives (Thomas VanArsdall)*
    - farmers want to produce safe food based on sound science (not headlines);.
    - government should ask only for what it needs as farmers are busy; and
    - in respect to change, urges pragmatic incrementalism.

- *United Fresh Fruit & Vegetable Association (John Aguirre)*
    - prefer government "guidance" to regulation; cooperation is key;
    - opposed to a single food safety agency as present food safety problems are not due to the lack of a single food agency;
    - does not support mandatory HACCP for all foods;
    - noted multiple instances of misguided responses by local officials to food contamination outbreaks (publicly blaming the wrong commodity), which led to producer and consumer harm; and
    - need more consumer education.

- *The United Egg Producers (Donald McNamara)*
    - egg producers answer to multiple agencies;
    - industry has programs to deal with risk and these good faith efforts work well;
    - need cooperative working relationships with government as a partner; and
    - need improved risk assessment.

Food Processors Panel
- *Grocery Manufacturers of America (Steve Ziller)*
    - US has safest food supply, but can do better;
    - change focus, not structure as will not make food safer to reorganize, but can make food safer if focus resources;
    - agencies need resources: scientists and dollars;
    - agencies must focus on real problems;
    - resist knee-jerk reactions, show leadership, less political science, and more real science; and
    - USDA continuous inspection uses scarce resources.

- *National Food Processors Association (Rhona Applebaum)*
  - US has perhaps the safest food supply;
  - FSIS has not always performed well, but HACCP is opening the process and becoming more transparent;
  - media has great power;
  - focus improvement on better cooperation among agencies;
  - focus on actual risks and put resources there;
  - need uniform approach across federal and state governments;
  - do not need single agency, just coordinate; and
  - most cost effective to fix current system.

- *American Meat Institute (James Hodges)*
  - current statute gives USDA no on-farm authority;
  - FSIS has greater resources then FDA, but fewer establishments to regulate as meat and poultry are the most regulated foods;
  - ability of FSIS to tailor efforts to risks is limited;
  - need more understanding of food production principles; and
  - FSIS should focus on verifying that food is safe rather than mandating how it gets safe, but not calling for suspension of continuous inspection.

- *International Dairy Food Association (Cary Frye)*
  - industry recognizes need to control pathogens;
  - HACCP should not be mandatory for dairy foods;
  - agencies need to be open minded, science based;
  - better state/federal cooperation needed; and
  - need uniformity in regulations.

- *National Fisheries Institute (Richard Gutting)*
  - present system works well;
  - seafood industry has partnerships with FDA and academia;
  - FDA is slow to respond to international seafood concerns;
  - loopholes in present system exist as sport fisherman deliver directly to restaurants (no HACCP program);
  - need science based information to make decisions; and
  - need more training and education.

  Summary: common themes of all panel members were the need for
  - **more public education, expanded government role at all levels;**
  - **increased communication and coordination among agencies;**
  - **more strengthening of research programs;**
  - **better coordination and transfer of technology; and**
  - **risk-based program with increased resources to accomplish the tasks, especially in FDA (resources).**

Ingredients and Packaging Panel

- *International Food Additive Council (Andrew Ebert)*
  - international harmonization is essential in order to facilitate US trade in the increasingly competitive world market; and
  - state and local regulations must be compatible with national regulations.

  Food Distributors International (John Block)
  - the US food system works because the food distribution industries are committed to a safe food supply; and
  - food distributors have developed their own HACCP system.

- *Society of the Plastic Industry, Inc. (Jerome Heckman)*
  - food packaging does not seem to be a public health or safety problem; and
    1997 FDA Modernization Act reduced the premarket notification system for food contact substances to 120 days.

  Summary: common themes of panel members were the need to
  - **increase reliance on academia, as the government science base has and is eroding;**
  - **give more responsibility to industry, with government providing knowledge for HACCP operations;**
  - **increase FDA funding to meet its statutory mandate;**
  - **eliminate or clarify and expedite FDA and FSIS duplication of efforts; and**
  - **coordination FDA and FSIS regulations for same product.**

Consumer Panel

- *Center for Science in the Public Interest (CSPI, Caroline Smith DeWaal) and Public Voice for Food and Health (Robert Hahn)*
  - both recommended a single food safety agency; and
  - food safety regulatory programs should not be linked with food marketing programs.

- *Consumers' Union (Mark Silbergeld)*
  - need "substantial consolidation" (which may be in the form of a single agency) to set standards, enforce the standards, and direct research;
  - both CDC and EPA should remain outside food safety regulatory mechanisms; and
  - need a single federal food safety research plan that is efficient and goal oriented.

Summary: common themes for all panel members were

- agencies sometimes have authority but lack political will to implement agreed upon solutions—example: *Salmonella* hazard in eggs;
- USDA and FDA need similar authority;
- need more outcome-oriented research programs;
- resources of agencies are not adequate to the task;
- agencies' responses and actions are not uniform;
- stakeholders often do not know who is in charge of a particular food safety issue, and federal employees frequently do not know either; and
- an ideal food safety system is coordinated, comprehensive, unified, hazard based, and streamlined. It has adequate funding and authority and strong educational programs.

Food Handlers Panel

- *Food Marketing Institute (Jill Hollingsworth)*
  - retailers have developed training programs for employees;
  - "Fight BAC" could be a model food safety program; and
  - need a single food safety voice as supermarket chains may have operations in multiple states and retailers deal with many federal, state, and local regulatory officials (one retailer reports to 88 different regulatory authorities).

- *National Restaurant Association (Judy Dausch)*
  - need to ensure that food safety agencies coordinate and harmonize their food safety standards;
  - development of national food safety standards should be based on risk and current available science;
  - need to increase funding for food handler training programs; and
  - need mandatory training and certification programs for state and local food safety inspectors.

- *United Food and Commercial Workers Union (Jackie Nowell)*
  - food handlers have a key role in influencing food safety;
  - food handlers often have low socioeconomic status;
  - food handler positions often provide no sick leave or other benefits, thus workers may come to work sick;
  - language barriers and high turnover limit the effectiveness of training programs; and
  - new regulations (HACCP) require time to implement, and have unanticipated effects on worker conditions (temperatures that are higher/lower than the comfort zone, exposure to cleaning agents).

State and Local Officials Panel

- *Association of Food and Drug Officials (Dan Smyly)*
  - – need to enhance effectiveness of federal, state, and local infrastructure currently in place rather than start over; and
  - – develop a blueprint for a vertically integrated national food system with input from all the major stakeholders.

- *National Association of State Departments of Agriculture (Richard Kirchhoff)*
  - – need to improve food safety education for consumers;
  - – HACCP system is a sound approach; however, parts of system (food animals) are left out of the regulatory scheme; and
  - – need more resources directed toward food imports.

- *Council of State and Territorial Epidemiologists (Dale Morse)*
  - – much public health activity is local;
  - – resources are in short supply and downsizing is occurring;
  - – need greater intra- and interagency coordination on major outbreaks;
  - – need to update technology; and
  - – allocate more resources to strengthening infrastructure for outbreak investigations.

Stakeholders in Policy Development Panel

- *Institute of Food Technologists (Bruce Stillings)*
  - – all food safety related functions should be placed in a single food safety agency;
  - – what works well: US has one of the safest food supplies in the world, regulating foods for biotechnology is science-based, and use of HACCP approach to inspection;
  - – food safety and public health must be primary purpose of food safety system, let industry address quality issues;
  - – food safety programs must encompass all aspects of food safety; and
  - – base food safety programs on risk assessment.

- *American Public Health Association (Eric Juzenas)*
  - – need single centralized, independent food safety agency to eliminate inconsistencies, gaps, and overlaps;
  - – what works well: good sanitation standards, food and nutritional supplement labeling, and food additives approvals;
  - – need mandatory recall authority;
  - – need to identify risks of imported foods;
  - – need food safety risk communication;

– need regulation of fruits and vegetables;
– need to address increasing resistance of pathogens to antimicrobials;
– need to address concerns about stress placed on animals during production;
– need improved surveillance system;
– need better coordination among state, local, and federal food safety programs;
– changes detrimental to national food safety program would be privatization of public health labs and too narrow a focus on a risk assessment; and
– if no agency has a primary responsibility for food safety, difficult to interest any agency in assisting with and focusing on food safety concerns.

Former Federal Government Food Safety Officials

• *Michael Taylor, former Deputy Commissioner for Policy of the Food and Drug Administration and Acting Administrator of the Food Safety and Inspection Service at US Department of Agriculture.*
    – the current reactive-based system dates back to beginning of the century;
    – shifting to science-based, preventive framework is the right track;
    – for new system to be successful, need to deploy resources in a new way, and to develop preventive strategies on system-wide basis;
    – current statutory and organization framework are obstacles to success due to fragmented nature of food safety research and misallocation of inspection resources;
    – need to pursue organizational change due to a present lack of clearly defined responsibility and accountability; and
    – need statutory reform.

• *Lester Crawford, former Administrator of the Food Safety and Inspection Service*
    – present system is disorganized;
    – *National Advisory Committee on Microbiological Specifications in Foods*, which involves four departments working effectively together, works well;
    – USDA conflicts associated with both promoting and regulating agriculture does not work well; and
    – no system for congressional oversight.

Summary: common themes by both **Michael Taylor and Lester Crawford**
- prevention of chronic illness and long-term public health concerns are different from food safety concerns;
- inspection and regulation should not be separated;
- resistance to change within FDA and USDA comes from both internal and external sources;
- any changes should be premised not on reducing staff and saving money but on re-deploying, modernizing and upgrading;
- problems with food safety research: not enough money, spread out from points of control and regulation, not a high priority in US research establishment, externally driven or investigator driven rather than a tool for achieving the food safety initiative;
- CDC should be a generator of fundamental knowledge; and
- need to address communication barriers among CDC, FDA, and FSIS.

Phase 3:   Open Forum
- *Food Animal Concerns Trust (FACT, Richard Wood)*
  - need a single food safety agency that has a single mission focusing on food safety, has clear roles and responsibilities, has regulatory authority joined with enforcement powers, and has farm-to-table regulatory responsibilities.

MEETING ON ENSURING SAFE FOOD
April 29–30, 1998
National Academy of Sciences Lecture Room

Agenda

Wednesday, April 29

8:30 am   **Welcome**
Allison Yates, Study Director
John Bailar, Chair, Committee

9:00 am   **International Perspectives for Ensuring Safe Food**
Ian Munro, CanTox, Inc.

9:45 am   **Organizational Strategies**
J. Clarence (Terry) Davies, Resources for the Future

10:30 am   Break
Ensuring Safe Food: Multi-Faceted Viewpoints

10:45 am   **Food Producers Panel Presentations**
Gary Weber, Animal Agriculture Coalition
Thomas VanArsdall, National Council of Farmer Cooperatives
John Aguirre, United Fresh Fruit and Vegetable Association
Donald McNamara, United Egg Producers

11:35 am   **Food Processors Panel Presentations**
Steve Ziller, Grocery Manufacturers of America
Rhona Applebaum, National Food Processors Association
James Hodges, American Meat Institute
Cary Frye, International Dairy Foods Association
Richard Gutting, National Fisheries Institute

12:35 pm   Lunch

1:30 pm   **Food Ingredients, Food Packaging, and Food Distribution Panel Presentations**
Andrew Ebert, International Food Additive Council
John Block, Food Distributors International
Jerome Heckman, The Society of the Plastics Industry, Inc.

2:10 pm   **Consumer Panel Presentations**
Caroline Smith DeWaal, Center for Science in the Public Interest
Mark Silbergeld, Consumers Union
Robert Hahn, Public Voice for Food and Health

2:50 pm   **Food Handlers Panel Presentations**
Jill Hollingsworth, Food Marketing Institute
Judy Dausch, National Restaurant Association
Jackie Nowell, United Food and Commercial Workers Union

3:30 pm   Break

3:45 pm   **Open Forum and Discussion**
Richard Wood, Food, Animals Concerns Trust

4:30 pm   Concluding Remarks, *John Bailar*

Thursday, April 30

8:30 am   **Welcome**
John Bailar

8:40 am   **State and Local Regulator Panel Presentations**
Dan Smyly, Association of Food and Drug Officials
*Richard Kirchhoff, National Association of State Departments of
    Agriculture*
Dale L. Morse, Council of State and Territorial Epidemiologists

9:20 am   **Stakeholders in Policy Development**
Bruce Stillings, Institute of Food Technologists
Eric Juzenas, American Public Health Association

10:00 am   Break

10:15 am   **Former Federal Government Food Safety Officials**
*Michael Taylor, former Deputy Commissioner for Policy of the Food and
    Drug Administration and former Administrator of the Food Safety and
    Inspection Service at the US Department of Agriculture*
*Lester Crawford, former Administrator of the Food Safety and Inspection
    Service at the US Department of Agriculture*

11:00 am   **Closing Remarks,** *John Bailar*

E

Federal Food Safety Budget Information

To assist the committee in determining the size and scope of the federal food safety budget, the committee asked the four major departments/agencies with responsibility for food safety to provide budget estimates for federal funds spent during the past four fiscal years. The agencies were requested to submit responses based on their involvement in one or more of five areas of federal food safety activity, as identified by the committee and emphasized in a National Food Safety Inititative (Appendix C). These areas are surveillance, inspection, risk assessment, research, and education. The responses of the agencies—the Department of Health and Human Services (DHHS), the United States Department of Agriculture (USDA), the Environmental Protection Agency (EPA), and the Department of Commerce—have been consolidated and appear in the table below. Copies of the committee questionnaire and each of the agency responses in full are available from the National Academy of Sciences' (NAS) public information file. Information on accessing these documents is available from the NAS website at **http://www.nas.edu.**

E

U.S. FOOD SAFETY BUDGETS (FY 1995–1998)

(in dollars)

	CDC[a]	NIH[b]	EPA[c]	FDA[d]	NMFS[e]	USDA[f]	Subtotal
Surveillance	not reported	not reported	not reported				
FY95	2,900,000			6,339,000		532,000	9,771,000
FY96	4,500,000			7,455,000		1,032,000	12,987,000
FY97	4,500,000			7,500,000		1,032,000	13,032,000
FY98	14,500,000			9,109,000		1,532,000	25,141,000
Inspection	not reported	not reported					
FY95			20,300,000	163,174,000	13,700,000	622,827,000	820,001,000
FY96			18,200,000	160,737,000	13,400,000	627,977,000	820,314,000
FY97			19,900,000	151,383,000	13,000,000	655,980,000	840,263,000
FY98			23,200,000	161,423,000	11,800,000	671,438,000	867,861,000
Risk Assessment	not reported	not reported					
FY95			91,100,000	6,339,000		5,887,000	103,326,000
FY96			107,400,000	7,455,000		6,885,000	121,740,000
FY97			133,100,000	7,500,000		8,272,000	148,872,000
FY98			126,700,000	9,109,000		7,598,000	143,407,000
Research	not reported						
FY95			13,100,000	22,913,000		47,812,000	83,825,000
FY96			12,200,000	22,266,000		47,333,000	81,799,000
FY97		49,799,000	19,000,000	21,977,000		53,557,000	144,333,000
FY98		52,873,000	32,000,000	25,632,000		60,348,000	170,853,000

Education	not reported	not reported	not reported				
FY95					12,698,000	5,638,000	18,336,000
FY96					13,771,000	5,651,000	19,422,000
FY97					15,137,000	5,390,000	20,527,000
FY98					17,308,000	5,523,000	22,831,000
Surveillance, Risk Assessment, Research, and Education							
FY95			7,900,000				7,900,000
FY96			7,800,000				7,800,000
FY97			7,300,000				7,300,000
FY98			6,700,000				6,700,000
TOTAL							
FY95	2,900,000	124,500,000	211,463,000		21,600,000	682,696,000	1,043,159,000
FY96	4,500,000	137,800,000	211,684,000		21,200,000	688,878,000	1,064,062,000
FY97	4,500,000	172,000,000	203,497,000	49,799,000	20,300,000	724,231,000	1,174,327,000
FY98	14,500,000	181,900,000	222,581,000	52,873,000	18,500,000	746,439,000	1,236,793,000

NOTE: For EPA there is no accounting system that separates food safety from other pesticide program activities. Therefore, the budget estimates provided here include a broader level of resources than just those directly related to food safety.

NOTE: NMFS has combined food safety surveillance, risk assessment, research, and education activities into a single category.

[a] Department of Health and Human Services, Division of Budget Formulation and Presentation. 1998. Written communication to committee.
[b] National Institutes of Health, Division of Nutrition Research Coordination and Nutritional Sciences Branch. 1998. Written Communication to Committee.
[c] Environmental Protection Agency, Office of Prevention, Pesticides, and Toxic Substances. 1998. Written communication to committee.
[d] Food and Drug Administration. 1998. Written communication to committee.
[e] United States Department of Commerce, National Marine Fisheries Service, Office of Sustainable Fisheries. 1998. Written communication to committee.
[f] United States Department of Agriculture. 1998. Written Communication to Committee.

F

Acknowledgments

The following individuals are among those who have provided assistance to the committee by providing oral testimony during the opening meetings, written comments, and/or written materials for the consideration by the committee.[*] Their assistance is greatly appreciated.

John Aguirre, United Fresh Fruit and Vegetable Association
Rhona Applebaum, National Food Producers Association
R. Thomas Van Arsdall, National Council of Farmer Cooperatives
Thomas Billy, Food Safety and Inspection Service
John R. Block, Food Distributors International
Leonard S. Bull, American Society of Animal Science (speaking only for himself)
Jean C. Buzby, Economic Research Service
Amie Chant, Sparks Companies
Jack L. Cooper, Food Industry Environmental Network
Lester M. Crawford, Georgetown University
Judith G. Dausch, National Restaurant Association
J. Clarence (Terry) Davies, Resources for the Future
Caroline Smith DeWaal, Center for Science in the Public Interest

[*] To review written comments submitted to the committee see the National Academy of Sciences' (NAS) public information file. Information on accessing these documents is available from the NAS website at **http://www.nas.edu**.

Richard J. Durbin, United States Senate
Andrew G. Ebert, International Food Additives Council
Jim Esselman, University of Virginia School of Law
John Farquhar, Food Marketing Institute
Vic Fazio, United States House of Representatives
Kirk Ferrell, National Pork Producers Council
Jeffrey K. Francer, John F. Kennedy School of Government, Harvard University
Michael A. Friedman, Food and Drug Administration
Cary P. Frye, International Dairy Foods Association
E. Spencer Garrett, National Marine Fisheries Service
Lynn R. Goldman, Environmental Protection Agency
Richard E. Gutting, Jr., National Fisheries Institute
Robert Hahn, Public Voice for Food and Health Policy
Betty Harden, Food and Drug Administration
Jerome H. Heckman, The Society of the Plastics Industry, Inc.
James H. Hodges, American Meat Institute
Jill Hollingsworth, Food Marketing Institute
Van Hubbard, National Institutes of Health
Karen Hulebak, Food and Drug Administration
Charles H. Jung, John F. Kennedy School of Government, Harvard University
Eileen Kennedy, United States Department of Agriculture
Richard Kirchoff, National Association of State Departments of Agriculture
Edward Knipling, United States Department of Agriculture
Joseph A. Levitt, Food and Drug Administration
Alan S. Levy, Food and Drug Administration
Jerold Mande, White House Office of Science and Technology Policy
Gary C. Matlock, National Marine Fisheries Service
Donald McNamara, United Egg Producers
Bruce C. Morehead, National Marine Fisheries Service
Ian C. Munro, CanTox, Inc.
Judy Nelson, Environmental Protection Agency
Jacqueline Nowell, United Food and Commercial Workers International Union
Janice Oliver, Food and Drug Administration
Soung Soo Pak, John F. Kennedy School of Government, Harvard University
Douglas Parson, Environmental Protection Agency
Morris Potter, Centers for Disease Control and Prevention
Donna Reifschneider, National Pork Producers Council
Richard Rominger, United States Department of Agriculture
William Schultz, Food and Drug Adminstration
Isi Sidiqqui, United States Department of Agriculture
Lisa Siegel, Food and Drug Administration
Mark Silbergeld, Consumers Union of U.S., Inc.
Dan S. Smyly, Association of Food and Drug Officials

Bruce R. Stillings, Institute of Food Technologists
Barbara S. Stowe, Human Sciences Institute, Inc.
Stephen Sundlof, Food and Drug Administration
Lyle P. Vogel, American Veterinary Medical Association
Donna Vogt, Congressional Research Service
Gary Weber, Animal Agriculture Coalition
Richard R. Wood, Food Animal Concerns Trust
Catherine E. Woteki, United States Department of Agriculture
David Wright, Harman and New Hope
Stephen A. Ziller, Grocery Manufacturers of America

G

Biographical Sketches

JOHN C. BAILAR III, M.D., Ph.D., (*Chair*), is Chair of the Department of Health Studies at the University of Chicago. He received his M.D. from Yale University and his Ph.D. from American University. His research involves quantitative health risk assessment with emphasis on the erosion of standards for scientific inference, pressures causing this erosion, and the ways the pressures might be reduced and quality preserved. He retired from the Commissioned Corps of the Public Health Service in 1980, served as a senior scientist at the Environmental Protection Agency from 1980 to 1982 and the Department of Health and Human Service's Office of Disease Prevention and Health Promotion from 1983 to 1992. In 1989, Dr. Bailar became a professor in the Department of Epidemiology and Biostatisics at McGill University and assumed his present position at the University of Chicago in 1995. He has served on numerous committees, including those of the National Academy of Sciences, American Medical Association, American Statistical Association, and Society for Risk Analysis. In 1993, Dr. Bailar was elected to membership in the Institute of Medicine. A well-known lecturer on science and public policy, Dr. Bailer is the author of over 200 scientific publications.

CAROLE A. BISOGNI, Ph.D., is Associate Professor and Associate Director for Academic Affairs in the Division of Nutritional Sciences at Cornell University, where she also holds joint appointments in the Institute for Food Science and the Institute for Comparative and Environmental Toxicology. She received her Ph.D. in Foods, Nutrition, and Microbiology from Cornell University. Her research interests include consumer food choices, risk communication, and public perceptions about food safety. She has published in scientific journals, written about food safety for the public, and worked with community nutritionists and other professionals in developing educational programs for adults and youths in different settings.

DAVID L. CALL, Ph.D., is former Dean of the College of Agriculture and Life Sciences at Cornell University, having held that position for 17 years before retiring in 1995. Throughout his career, Dr. Call's research has focused on analyses of government food and nutrition programs, identification and analysis of factors causing changes in nutrition and food consumption, and international economic and development issues. He has served on numerous national advisory panels, including the National Advisory Committee to the Commissioner of the Food and Drug Administration; the Office of Technology Assessment Food Advisory Panel; and the White House Conference on Food, Nutrition, and Health. Dr. Call is a former member of the Institute of Medicine's Food and Nutrition Board and the 1978 National Academy of Sciences Committee for a Study on Food Safety and Food Safety Policy, and he is a former chair of the National Academy of Sciences Committee on Technological Options to Improve the Nutritional Attributes of Animal Products. Having served as a member of the national-level Board of Trustees for the Food Safety Council from 1979 through 1982, he has addressed food safety issues for many years. He has served at the state and local levels on numerous commissions dealing with social and economic aspects of food and nutrition priorities. Dr. Call received his B.S., M.S., and Ph.D. in agricultural economics from Cornell University and has published widely on food systems and consumer issues. He is currently a Director of The Seneca Foods Corporation and of Cayuga Aquacultures and is a Trustee of The Mutual of New York Insurance Company.

MARSHA N. COHEN, J.D., is Professor of Law at Hastings College of the Law, University of California, where she has been since 1976. She received her undergraduate degree from Smith College and a J.D. from Harvard Law School. Professor Cohen teaches courses in administrative law and torts. She represents the interest of consumers on the Institute of Medicine's Food Forum and was a member of its Committee on State Food Labeling. Presently, she is a consultant to the Food Advisory Committee of the Food and Drug Administration and has consulted extensively on food safety issues for Consumers Union. Professor Cohen was a member of the Keystone National Policy Dialogue on Food, Nutrition, and Health. She is the co-author of a text on pharmacy law.

MICHAEL P. DOYLE, Ph.D., is Regents Professor of Food Microbiology, Director of the Center for Food Safety and Quality Enhancement, and Head of the Department of Food Science and Technology at the University of Georgia. He is an active researcher in the area of foodborne bacterial pathogens and works closely with the food industry on issues related to the microbiological safety of foods. Dr. Doyle's research focuses on the study of the mechanisms of pathogenicity, the development of methods for pathogen detection, and the identification of means to control or eliminate pathogens from foods. He received his Ph.D. in food microbiology from the University of Wisconsin. He was with Ralston Purina Company from 1977 to 1980 and on the faculty at the University of Wisconsin from 1980 until 1991. He is a currently a member of the Institute of Medicine's Food Forum and is a past member of the Food and Nutrition Board and Board on Agriculture's Panel on Animal Health and Veterinary Medicine. In addition, Dr. Doyle serves on the Board of Trustees and Executive Committee of the International Life Sciences Institute-North America, the Scientific Advisory Council of The Refrigeration Research and Education Foundation, and the International Commission on Microbiological Specifications for Foods, and he is a consultant to several food companies on food safety-related issues. He has published more than 200 scientific articles as well as being editor of two authoritative books: *Foodborne Bacterial Pathogens* and *Food Microbiology: Fundamentals and Frontiers.*

DELIA A. HAMMOCK, M.S., R.D., has been Associate Director of the Good Housekeeping Institute for the past 10 years. She serves as the Institute spokesperson on nutrition issues, frequently addressing professional and trade associations at state and national conventions and appearing on public media. She has a dual role in the Institute: (1) she functions as the in-house expert on nutrition and writes monthly features on diet, nutrition, and food issues for *Good Housekeeping* magazine and (2) she reviews all food advertisements and products for acceptability under *Good Housekeeping*'s Consumer Warranty. She is a registered dietitian and holds an M.S. in nutrition from Boston University. Before her position at the magazine, she was a food and nutrition communications specialist, with clients including the New York Heart Association, Metropolitan Life Insurance Company, and several national magazines. From 1981 to 1986 she was an adjunct instructor in the Department of Nutrition at New York University. From 1978 to 1984 she served as pediatric nutrition specialist at New York University Medical Center and was a clinical nutritionist at New York Hospital from 1975 to 1977. Since 1990, Ms. Hammock has provided numerous public presentations on the consumer's view of food safety issues.

LONNIE KING, D.V.M., is currently Dean of the College of Veterinary Medicine at Michigan State University. He was Administrator of the Animal and Plant Health Inspection Service of the U.S. Department of Agriculture from 1992 to 1996. Prior to this, he served as the agency's Associate Administrator and Deputy Administrator for Veterinary Services. Dr. King was in private practice before his government career. His other experiences include work as a field veterinary medical officer, station epidemiologist, and staff assignments involving Emergency Programs and Animal Health Information. He has also directed the American Veterinary Medical Association's Office of Governmental Relations and is boarded in the American College of Veterinary Preventive Medicine. He received his B.S. and D.V.M. from the Ohio State University and holds an M.S. in epidemiology from the University of Minnesota and an M.S. in public administration from American University.

GILBERT A. LEVEILLE, Ph.D., recently retired from his position as Vice President, Research and Technical Services, with Nabisco, Inc., where he was responsible for fundamental science, analytical services, and extrusion research. He continues to have a consulting relationship with Nabisco and consults with other companies, including Monsanto, McNeil Consumer Products, Cultor, and Safety Associates. He received his Ph.D. from Rutgers University. Previously, Dr. Leveille was Professor and Chairman of the Department of Food Science and Human Nutrition at Michigan State University and was Director of Nutrition and Health Sciences at General Foods Corporation. He is a past president of the Institute of Food Technologists and of the American Society for Clinical Nutrition and is a member of numerous other professional organizations. Dr. Leveille currently serves on the FDA Science Advisory Board and on the Board of Directors of the Riley Memorial Foundation. He lectures widely and has published more than 300 scientific papers and several books.

RICHARD A. MERRILL, LL.B., is Daniel Caplin Professor of Law at the University of Virginia School of Law, where he has been since 1969, and is of Counsel to the Washington, D.C., law firm of Covington & Burling. Professor Merrill earned his A.B. at Columbia College and his LL.B. at Columbia University School of Law. He also received a B.A. and an M.A. from Oxford University, where he was a Rhodes Scholar. From 1975 to 1977, he was Chief Counsel of the Food and Drug Administration. Professor Merrill teaches courses in food and drug law, administrative law, and environmental law. He has served as a member of several committees of the National Academy of Sciences and was elected to membership in its Institute of Medicine in 1978. He has been a consultant on food safety issues to the former Office of Technology Assessment of the Congress and the White House Office of Science and Technology Policy. Professor Merrill is a member of the American Law Institute and a fellow of the Virginia Law Foundation. He is General Counsel to the Chemical Industry Institute of Technology and is on the Board of the Health and Environmental Sciences Institute, an affiliate of the International Life Sciences Institute. He is the author of law school texts as well as numerous articles on food and drug law and administrative law.

SANFORD A. MILLER, Ph.D., is Dean of the Graduate School of Biomedical Sciences and Professor in the Departments of Biochemistry and Medicine at the University of Texas Health Science Center at San Antonio. He is the former Director of the Center for Food Safety and Applied Nutrition at the Food and Drug Administration. Previously, he was a Professor of Nutritional Biochemistry at the Massachusetts Institute of Technology. Dr. Miller has served on many national and international government and professional society advisory committees, including the Federation of American Societies for Experimental Biology Expert Committee on GRAS Substances, the National Advisory Environmental Health Sciences Council of NIH, the Institute of Medicine's Food and Nutrition Board and Food Forum, the Joint FAO/WHO Expert Advisory Panel on Food Safety (Chair), and the Joint FAO/WHO Expert Consultation on the Application of Risk Analysis to Food Standard Issues (Chair). Dr. Miller also serves as a consultant to Nabisco Foods; Source Foods; and Patton, Boggs, and Blow and as an advisor to Nestle and the International Advisory Council of the Monell Chemical Senses Center. He has written more than 200 scientific publications. Dr. Miller received his M.S. and Ph.D. in physiology and biochemistry from Rutgers University.

HARLEY W. MOON, Ph.D., D.V.M., is F.K. Ramsey Chair of Veterinary Medicine at Iowa State University. He has been a member of the National Academy of Sciences since 1991. Dr. Moon is most widely recognized for his contributions to the basic understanding of intestinal diseases of humans and animals. His expertise includes the development of vaccines for preventing *E. coli* infection in farm animals, livestock disease eradication, infectious diseases affecting humans and animals, and prevention of edema disease in swine with genetically modified vaccines. Dr. Moon has served on numerous advisory committees, including the World Health Organization's Expert Panel on Enteropathogenic *E. coli* and Working Group on Immunology and Vaccine Development for Bacterial Enteric Infections, the Department of Agriculture's Task Force on Scrapie and Bovine Spongiform Encephalopathy, Pioneer Hi-Bred International's Institutional Biosafety Committee, and Council for Agricultural Science and Technology Task Force on Antibiotics in Animal Feeds. He presently serves as a consultant to Agricultural Technology Partners, L.P., and owns and manages a farm in Iowa. His scientific publications number in excess of 200, with numerous book chapters on aspects of infectious disease. Before his current position, Dr. Moon was director of the Plum Island and National Animal Disease Centers, ARS/USDA, and professor in the Department of Veterinary Pathology at Ohio State University. He received his B.S., D.V.M., and Ph.D. at the University of Minnesota.

MICHAEL T. OSTERHOLM, Ph.D., is State Epidemiologist and Chief, Acute Disease Epidemiology Section, Minnesota Department of Health. He is also an adjunct professor in the Division of Epidemiology, School of Public Health, University of Minnesota. Dr. Osterholm is considered a leader in the area of infectious disease epidemiology. He has led numerous investigations of infectious disease outbreaks, including foodborne diseases, and is the author of more than 160 papers and 12 book chapters regarding infectious disease epidemiology. Dr. Osterholm is past president of the Council of State and Territorial Epidemiologists. He is a current member of the National Advisory Committee on the Microbiological Criteria for Food. He participates in the NAS IOM Forum on Emerging Infectious Diseases and recently served on the CDC Board of Scientific Counselors. He chairs the Committee on Public Health and serves on the Public and Scientific Affairs Board, the Task Force on Biological Weapons, and the Task Force on Antibiotic Resistance of the American Society for Microbiology and chairs the Emerging Infections Committee of the Infectious Diseases Society of America. Dr. Osterholm is a frequent consultant to NIH, FDA, and CDC and currently serves as a principal investigator to the CDC Emerging Infections Program.

THOMAS D. TRAUTMAN, Ph.D., is Principal Scientist, Toxicology and Regulatory Affairs, for General Mills, where he has been for 20 years. He received his Ph.D. in Comparative Pharmacology and Toxicology from the University of California at Davis. Dr. Trautman has been actively involved in food industry efforts to address numerous food safety and regulatory issues, including the safety of food and color additives, pesticide residues, food allergy, packaging and other indirect additives, and various aspects of current and emerging risk assessment methodologies. He is a Diplomate of the American Board of Toxicology and is Chair of the Food Safety Section of the Society of Toxicology. Dr. Trautman is a former member of the National Academy of Sciences Board on Agriculture, is a member and former Chair of the Toxicology and Safety Evaluation Division of the Institute of Food Technologists, and was the founding Chair of the Residue Committee of the International Life Sciences Institute.